SAVE YOUR HANDS!

Injury Prevention for Massage Therapists

Lauriann Greene, L.M.P.

Edited by Robert A. Greene, M.D.
Clinical Assistant Professor
University of Rochester School of Medicine

D0126286

Infinity Press

8 7 6 5 4 3

Published by Infinity Press
P.O. Box 17883, Seattle, WA 98107-1883, USA.

Manufactured in the United States of America.

Edited by Robert A. Greene, M.D.
Cover design by Jackie A. Phillips, Jackie Philips Design
Photography by Steve Meltzer
Medical Illustrations by Christine Shafner, K.E. Sweeney Illustration Studio
Design by Fred Wert, Infinity Press

Library of Congress Cataloging-in-Publication Data:

Greene, Lauriann, 1960 -
        Save Your Hands!
        Bibilography: p. 157
        Includes index
        1. Massage, therapeutic 2. Health 3. Body, human
ISBN 1-883195-03-9

Library of Congress Catalog Number 95-80459

 Printed on 85% recycled paper.

Preface

I learned about massage-related injury the hard way: by personal experience. I had always been a physically inactive, delicately-built person with little natural strength or endurance. I decided to become a massage therapist after ten years spent sitting at a desk as an arts administrator. When I began my massage training, I told myself I would start working out to get stronger. Between going to school and working part-time, I could never find the time to go to the gym. In my second term at school, I started feeling twinges of pain in my right wrist whenever I did certain techniques. I wasn't sure what these twinges meant or what was causing them, so I kept on massaging and doing those same techniques. The pain continued and worsened. I tried icing my wrist, and resting during a two-week school break, both of which brought some relief.

When the next term began, I signed up for a seven-week externship at a medical clinic. Up to that point, I had been giving only one or two massages per week. Suddenly, I was giving eight to twelve massages per day, two days per week at the clinic, with little or no break between sessions. The pain returned, along with stiffness and tightness in my hands and forearms. I knew I needed to stop doing so many massages, but the clinic receptionist had already scheduled appointments for me through the end of my externship. I felt pressured to continue; after all, how could I disappoint the patients, the doctors who referred them to me, and the school that would judge my performance in the program? By the end of the seven weeks, I was in constant pain in both my wrists and both my arms, and I was scared. It was no longer only massage that produced the pain. Everything seemed to make my wrists hurt: opening a door, turning a faucet, even brushing my teeth was painful. I finally saw a physician, who diagnosed my condition as a severe repetitive stress injury. The combination of lack of strength and doing an unnatural motion over and over had caused me to overstress and damage the tissues of my wrists. I started a course of occupational and physical therapy that lasted seven months.

I made it through the end of my professional licensing course by doing as few massages as I could get away with. I took my boards, passed, and got my license. On the advice of my doctor and physical therapist, I completely stopped doing massage so my injury could heal. I did not give a massage again for over a year. My massage career was over before it had begun.

My injury affected every aspect of my life. I worried that I would lose my ability to make a living, since I could barely use my hands without pain. The first two weeks after I stopped doing massage, I had to ask a friend to come live with me and do manual tasks such as opening jars and turning faucets, and even holding the blow dryer for me as I dried my hair. I was depressed and angry, and the constant pain in my wrists made me feel even worse. A kind psychotherapist helped me deal with the emotional pain, but it took another year before my hands felt anywhere near normal again.

As I dealt with my injury, I began to realize that it was part of a bigger problem, one that affected not just me, but all massage therapists. Other students in my school were getting symptoms of injury starting as early as two months into the program. Every massage therapist who saw me with splints on my wrists immediately started relating his or her experience with massage-related injury. It seemed that almost everyone I met who did massage on a regular basis had at some time experienced pain or injury in their upper extremities.

As I read texts on massage, it struck me that the emphasis was always on ensuring the comfort and safety of the client, not the practitioner. Few massage texts even brought up the subject of injury from doing massage. If they did, it was to state simply that massage therapists tend to get arthritis in their hands and wrists after a while, and to recommend rest if the therapist began to feel symptoms of injury. It was clear that this problem was not being addressed adequately in the profession. How could we effectively promote health and well-being for our clients while we were getting hurt ourselves? All the recent information in the news about repetitive stress injuries, carpal tunnel syndrome, etc., was beginning to open the eyes of the general public to the physical hazards of hand-intensive occupations. I felt it was time for someone in the massage field to start offering massage students and professionals practical information that could help them save their most valuable working tool: their hands.

Since I could no longer give hands-on massages, I decided to use my training to research and write about occupation-related upper extremity injury. I published a magazine article on musicians' injuries (I'm a musician myself), and was shocked to learn in my research that repetitive stress injuries are epidemic among instrumentalists. I felt even more motivated to design an injury-prevention workshop for massage therapists. I based the "Save Your Hands!" workshop on consultations and studies with some of my own physical therapists, as well as the research I had done on the article. With the help and encouragement of my alma mater, Seattle Massage School, I began teaching these workshops regularly at its three campuses. I have also taught "Save Your Hands!" workshops at massage schools and studios in Eastern Washington; Vancouver, British Columbia; Boulder, Colorado; and several locations in New York State.

Over the past two and one half years, hundreds of students and licensed massage practitioners have taken the workshop. They have told me that the information and techniques I taught helped them feel that they could protect their investment in this challenging career by taking care of themselves. Seeing so many therapists helped me develop a profile of the kind of symptoms massage therapists experience and the kinds of injuries they sustain in relation to their work. It also confirmed for me how common and devastating these injuries are. Many of the therapists I saw were already injured, and were struggling to get through school or keep their practices going through the pain. Although I was doing one workshop per month in different locations, I realized that there were still thousands of massage therapists I would never reach. I wanted to make sure that every massage student and therapist could have access to this important information, and the best way to accomplish my goal was to write this book, based on the workshop.

I know how devastating it can be to have your massage career, and your life, interrupted by injury. In my workshops, I joke with my students that I have made myself the "poster child" for massage-related hand and arm injury: imagine a picture of a former massage therapist with splints on both hands and the caption, "Don't let this happen to you. Together, we can make sure it never happens again!" I hope this book is the first step in making that wish a reality.

Lauriann Greene, L.M.P.

Seattle, Washington, 1995

Acknowledgements

This book could not have been written without the kind assistance of colleagues, friends and family. I would like to particularly thank:

All of the "Save Your Hands!" workshop participants, for asking so many great questions, and for sharing their experiences and stress-reducing techniques with me. I wish you all long, healthy, fulfilling massage careers!

My colleagues in the massage profession: Diana Thompson, for her inspiring teaching, empathy as a fellow author, and her insightful editing; Clint Chandler for encouraging me to develop and teach the workshop; Dawn Schmidt, Greg Bolton and Stan Saltzberg of Seattle Massage School for caring enough about their students to let me teach the "Save Your Hands" workshops at their school; and Rafael Tuberan and David Palmer for their thoughtful review of the manuscript.

My collaborators on this project: Infinity Press for their good humor, generosity, support, and belief in my abilities; Steve Meltzer for the wonderful photos and for continuing to be my photographic collaborator; and Jason Atlas and Melissa Page for their time and patience as models.

Two gifted physical therapists who deepened my understanding of the complexities of upper extremity injury and provided invaluable information for the exercise and treatment portions of the book: Craig London, who also helped me recover from my own injury; and Ellen Roth, who also hooked me up with the wonderful folks at Infinity Press.

Most of all, I would like to thank my brother, Dr. Robert A. Greene, for his phenomenal knowledge and remarkable editing skills that transformed this book, as well as his support, encouragement, and love; Dr. Susan Presberg-Greene for her good advice and moral support; my wonderful friends, especially Susan Schreiber, PT, Dr. Kristen Anderson, Angelica Arenas, Richard Vitzhum, and Catherine Hurd; and my parents, Claire and David Greene, who have always made me feel that I could do anything I put my mind to, and who have been there for me through it all.

Disclaimer

The purpose of this book is to provide basic information for massage therapists on the subject of occupation-related injury in order to increase their awareness of this issue. This book does not offer medical advice to the reader, and is not intended as a replacement or substitute for appropriate health care and treatment. Readers who experience any signs or symptoms of injury have the resonsiblitity to seek professional medical advice and treatment.

Injury is a complex subject. The author and publisher have made considerable efforts to ensure the accuracy of the information provided herein. However, there may be mistakes or typographical errors in the contents of the book. Therefore, this book should be used as a general text, and is by no means to be considered the definitive or sole source of information on this subject. The techniques and recommendations included in the book are meant as general suggestions. They are not to be construed as specific directions for any one reader, and may need to be adapted to fit the individual's body and work situation. The reader is encouraged to refer to other books on the subject for further edification; a list of suggested additional reading is included in the Bibliography.

The author and publisher of this book have no liability or responsibility for any loss or damage incurred to any person or entity caused or alleged to be caused, either directly or indirectly, by any information presented in this book.

If you do not wish to be bound by the above, you may return this book to the publisher for a full refund.

Table of Contents

Introduction

Professional massage therapists and massage students get injured from giving massages. Repetitive stress injuries are an occupational hazard for massage therapists, just as they are for computer operators and musicians. The information provided in this book will help you take the necessary steps to protect your hands and your massage career.

Save Your Hands! is meant to be a source book for all massage therapists, from beginning students to experienced professionals. The information presented here will be most applicable to the large majority of students and practitioners who do the types of massage that involve strenuous use of the hands and/or techniques that call for endurance and strength to manipulate the muscles and joints (such as Swedish or Deep Tissue Massage). However, the information, suggestions, and techniques in this book can help *any bodyworker* have a long, healthy, injury-free career.

Massage students: You will learn how and why injury happens, information that will help you protect your own health and better understand your clients' complaints. You will also learn how to develop stress-reducing massage habits while you are still in school, so you will be ready for the demands of your new career. Massage-related injury is common among massage students: protect your investment in this challenging career by learning as early as possible how to stay healthy as you work!

Professional massage therapists: You will find an organized, concise approach to occupation-related upper extremity injury that will help you understand and prevent injury. It is the rare massage practitioner who can massage for years without ever developing any symptoms of injury or impending injury. You can protect your career by learning as much about injury as possible, and finding ways to put less stress on your arms and hands. Your increased understanding of repetitive stress injuries will also be invaluable in treating your clients.

Massage educators or massage school administrators: You also will find a great deal of information in this book that is pertinent to your work. School is the ideal place to introduce injury prevention concepts and techniques. After all, a massage therapist's first perceptions about massage as a profession are often developed when she or he is a student. Teaching students to protect their own health is perhaps the most important service we can offer as educators. With increased awareness of massage-related injury, it is the author's hope that schools will augment their efforts to train students about this important issue. Appendix II contains suggestions and recommendations for approaches to teaching injury prevention, as well as curriculum development. Since information in this book can easily be translated to other repetitive stress injuries, it can also be used as an adjunct text to a massage school's clinical treatment curriculum.

To prevent massage-related injury, you need to integrate the two things that make you who you are: your mind and your body. Your mind needs information, so you can make informed decisions about creating a healthy career in massage. This information comes partially from books like this one. The rest comes from your own body. Developing body awareness, a heightened consciousness of your physical state, will enable you to listen and respond to your body, and keep it injury-free. *Save Your Hands!* helps you achieve this integration by giving you:

• **A method of thinking about injury**. You need to know not only *that* massage therapists get injured, but *why* they get injured. This information can help you figure out what caused your injury so you can avoid doing it again. Musculoskeletal injury is a very complex subject. One book cannot teach you everything there is to know about injury. This book will give you an organized way of *thinking* about injury. After reading *Save Your Hands!*, you will be able to make some basic assumptions and deductions when you encounter injury that will enable you to give, or seek, better treatment. Although the injuries included here are discussed in terms of massage therapists, they are also quite common in the general population, which includes your clients. Reading this book will therefore enhance your practice as well as your knowledge.

• **Ways to help you develop body awareness.** How does your body respond to doing massage? Are you comfortable as you work? Are there things about your own body that could make you more susceptible to injury? *Save Your Hands!* will help you think about your body in new ways, giving you the heightened awareness you need to protect yourself from injury.

• **A stress-reducing way of doing massage.** There are many ways of doing hands-on work. *Save Your Hands!* offers you ways to adapt your techniques to make them easier on your hands and arms.

They will help you feel comfortable and relaxed as you massage; after all, your work should be pleasant and invigorating, not torturous!

• **Treatment options**. If you are already experiencing symptoms, or if you develop symptoms at any point in your career, you will need to know all you can about effective treatment methods. This book includes a thorough discussion of available treatment options, as well as guidelines for finding professional health care and dealing with the emotional fallout of injury.

Save Your Hands! concentrates on injuries of the upper extremity. Massage therapists do experience injury to other parts of the body as a result of giving massages, especially the back. But since doing massage most commonly injures the upper extremity, I have chosen to focus on injury to the fingers/hand, wrist, forearm, elbow, upper arm, and shoulder girdle (the complex of the humerus and the scapula). Many of the general concepts about injury and self-care presented in the book can be applied to other parts of the body as well.

This book is based on extensive research on occupation-related upper extremity injury, the anecdotal experiences of my workshop attendees and massage colleagues, private consultations with injured massage students and professionals, and my own experience with massage-caused injury. Unfortunately, there is very little literature on the topic of massage-related injury at this time. The chapter on treatment discusses extensively those modalities commonly accepted as effective treatments for these kinds of injuries. There are many alternative treatment options available as well. I encourage you to find out as much as you can about all kinds of treatment, and try the ones you feel might be helpful.

For your reference, a glossary of terms used in the book is included, as well as an index to help you find specific topics of interest, and a bibliography that will direct you to sources of further information on the subject. There is also a short self-quiz you can take to increase your injury self-awareness.

The risk of occupation-related injury is an ever-present threat for massage therapists. With proper attention and care, you can prevent injury from interfering with your work and your life. Knowledge and awareness are very empowering tools. Use them in your work every day, and you *will* be able to save your hands!

1

Making a Healthy Career in Massage

Massage is one of the great pleasures of life. Its benefits as a healing art have been known for thousands of years. Most people like to receive massage, and many people like giving them. Massage can be both a simple, direct means of positive communication and an effective therapeutic modality. For all these reasons and more, the idea of making a career in massage is very appealing to many people.

In the United States, massage has enjoyed a renaissance in the past thirty years. Before the sixties, massage had become a rarefied service to which few people had access. Athletes could get a rubdown after a game, the rich could indulge in luxurious pampering at expensive spas, and men could pay for sensual massage in "massage parlors." In the more open, liberated atmosphere of the sixties, people became more body conscious, sensuality was more acceptable, and alternative healing methods became more accessible. The general public became willing to take a new look at massage, and slowly rediscovered that it could be a legitimate form of healing and a natural, wholesome, enjoyable experience.

Now massage is finally beginning to be accepted not only by the public, but also by the medical community and insurance companies, as a bona fide health care modality. Massage schools are increasing in number (there are now more than 400 in the U.S. and Canada) and students are flocking to them with hopes of creating a meaningful, profitable career for themselves.

While those in the profession have worked hard to gain this acceptance, it came with a price. In becoming mainstream, massage therapy had to adapt to society's still somewhat narrow health care expectations. It had to align itself with traditional Western allopathic medicine to some degree, and adopt the medical model of treatment aimed at fixing a particular problem with a particular technique. Much of the pressure comes from insurance companies and worker's compensation, who will not reimburse for massage unless they see clear, quantifiable results for a specific diagnosis using recognized and accepted massage techniques. The range of massage techniques that fit into this category of "recognized and accepted" is still quite small, limited mostly to pressure-intensive techniques like deep tissue and trigger point work. Massage therapists hoping to be paid by these sources had to gear their practices to this model, and "treatment massage" became the popular way to practice.

In response to the demand for massage therapists who could do the kind of treatment work that would be reimbursed by insurance, massage schools began to incorporate more clinical treatment into their curricula. The schools understandably want to prepare their students for the kind of work that will be required of them as professionals. They began to make a distinction between those techniques that could be part of "relaxation massage" and those that were used for "treatment massage." Typically, schools taught students that "relaxation" techniques were traditional Swedish movements that encompassed the whole body with broad, large, sweeping movements. "Treatment" techniques pinpointed smaller areas of injury using deep pressure, and finer, repetitive movements. Often therapists needed to use a small part of their hand, often a thumb, as a tool to get at these tiny problem spots. Unfortunately, this emphasis on small, repetitive motions and spot work proved to be potentially harmful for the students. What became known as "treatment massage" ended up being much harder on the therapist's hands than "relaxation massage" ever was.

Added to this problem is the ever-increasing demand for massage services. While the increase in popularity of massage among the general public has been a welcome occurrence, with it comes increased pressure on massage practitioners to do more and more massages. Massage therapists naturally want to get as much work as possible so they can make a good living by doing massage. However, there is a new danger of therapists over-booking themselves and putting unrealistic demands on their bodies. Therapists working in clinics and spas find a new pressure has been put on them to do more massage in shorter amounts of time. When the number of massages a practitioner gives increases dramatically, and the work they are doing becomes more difficult at the same time, injury becomes an ever-present risk.

The "masseuses and masseurs" of the past worked hard in hotels, spas and clubs. Certainly some of them got injured from their work. There was not, however, the pressure to produce, nor the emphasis on treatment. In massage clinics, health clubs, and chiropractic offices, massage therapists now work long hours, with little time between sessions, doing mostly treatment work. Giving four or five Swedish relaxation massages in a day is challenging, but giving the same number of "treatment" massages in the same amount of time is hazardous. The result has been an epidemic of repetitive stress injuries among massage therapists.

Unfortunately, the definition of what constitutes "treatment" in massage has become too narrow, both for massage therapists and for the public, insurance companies, and other health care providers. Treatment has more to do with *intent* and *focus* than on any specific technique. One of the beauties of massage is its ability to be both relaxing and therapeutic *at the same time*. Any massage technique can be used to treat a specific complaint if treatment is the therapist's goal in using that technique. For this reason, many clients receive therapeutic benefits from massage techniques as diverse as energy work, polarity, Trager movement therapy, and craniosacral work. The ability to create a therapeutic effect is one of the most subtle aspects of massage, a skill that takes experience and maturity to attain. Until they have practiced long enough to acquire this skill, massage therapists rely on technique. When that technique is overly stressful to their bodies, they get hurt.

There is no question that massage therapists practicing today have to deal with many new and challenging pressures. Today's massage therapists need to be tougher, better trained, in better physical condition, and more careful in their work than ever before if they are going to withstand the demands of this changing profession. Massage professionals need to become massage "athletes."

Becoming a Massage Athlete

There is good news and bad news about doing massage.

First, the bad news: massage is very hard on your hands and upper extremities. Except for those massage therapists who do mostly very light techniques (e.g. energy balancing or craniosacral work), most practitioners will experience some kind of injury or pain syndrome at some point in their careers as a result of giving massages. *Anyone* who works intensively with his or her hands, like carpenters, cashiers, musicians, or computer operators, is prone to upper extremity injury, since the intensity of this work is more than most bodies can take. The arms and hands, with their small muscles, bones and ligaments, just were not designed to withstand this type of work for extended periods of time.

Now the good news: there is a great deal you can do to protect yourself from this kind of injury. The key is to think of yourself as an athlete. Just like a runner or a baseball player, you are doing intense, physical work that requires skill, strength, and endurance. For all athletes, the parts of the body most used in their sport are the ones most likely to become injured. For baseball pitchers it is the elbow and shoulder, for runners it is the knees and legs. The massage "athlete" uses her upper extremity (including the shoulder girdle) extensively in her work, and it is this part of her body that is most prone to injury.

Like any other athlete, the massage therapist needs to train, stay in good physical condition, and "bench" herself when she is injured to allow enough time for healing. An athlete is very aware of her own body, since it is her tool for doing her job. In contrast, since massage therapists tend to think of themselves more as healers or caregivers, they focus on thinking about how to treat the client, not on the physical process by which they accomplish the treatment. They split off the mind from the body, the intellectual process from the physical work. By concentrating so much more on the intellectual process than the physical one, massage therapists end up discounting or ignoring the way their bodies are responding to (or suffering from) the intense work they are doing. In general, the massage therapist's *own* body is the last thing on his mind when he is giving a massage.

Body Awareness - Your Best Protection Against Injury

The best way to combat this split between the mind and body is to develop body awareness. Body awareness is a consciousness of your body's strengths and weaknesses, advantages and limitations. This consciousness makes you more attentive to the signals your body sends you as you give a massage. We all have physical strengths and weaknesses; there is no value judgment implied here. Having a weak point does not make you a bad therapist, just as having a strength does not make you a good one. Awareness allows you to accentuate your best attributes while minimizing the effect of your less-than-optimum ones on your work and your health. One of the great benefits of receiving massage is, in fact, developing greater body awareness. During a massage, the client has an opportunity to focus on his body's reactions to touch. Helping your clients develop body awareness is a valuable service that will help them stay healthy. Awareness helps you stay in tune with your body, so you can respond promptly to symptoms and keep yourself from becoming injured.

Making Informed Choices about Your Massage Career

Once you have developed awareness of your body's strengths and weaknesses, you will be better able to choose the kind of massage career you should pursue. Having a realistic view of how well your body is adapted to performing the physical work of giving massages will help you make an informed decision.

If you choose to pursue a full-time career in massage, you will need to maintain a high level of physical fitness in order to stay healthy. You will need to build upper body strength and develop endurance. If you have limited upper body strength and are not in good condition to begin with, this process may take a while. Some people who are out-of-shape when they begin their massage education assume that they will develop strength and endurance as they go along in school simply from doing massage. The problem is that even in your first term of school, you will be asked to do techniques that call for a certain amount of strength and endurance. You will also be using muscles that you may not often use in everyday life. The demands placed on you may increase faster than your level of fitness. Even if you make it through school without becoming injured, it is unlikely that you will be able to sustain a full-time career unless you make a commitment to start working out.

It is important to realize that a full-time massage career is not for everyone, just as not everyone is capable of being a professional athlete or musician. If you do not enjoy doing physically demanding work or exercise, you probably will not do well in a massage career that emphasizes deep work using a great deal of pressure.

Body type also influences your suitability for a given profession. Football players tend to be big and stocky, because they need the extra bulk to make good tackles. Basketball players are usually tall, because they need the height to sink the ball in the basket. Basketball players who are not very tall, or football players who are not very big, have to compensate for their deficiencies in other ways, for example by being very fast and agile. The stereotypical massage therapist used to be a person with big, strong hands and a broad, muscular build. In fact, persons with that kind of physique and natural strength *do* have an easier time giving a massage without getting injured. If you are not built like that, you will have to compensate for it in some other way.

You have many options if you decide that a full-time massage career is not a realistic goal for you. One option is a part-time career in massage. Find a number of massages per week that feels comfortable for you and limit yourself to those massages. Then work on your upper body strength. In time, you may find that you do develop enough strength to slowly increase the number of massages you do per week. It is perfectly legitimate to have a part-time practice, or to do massage as a sideline, or to give massages to friends and loved ones exclusively.

You also may want to consider other types of bodywork that do not take as much strength and physical effort. Many people find specialties like Reiki, energy balancing, polarity therapy, Feldenkrais, Trager, and craniosacral treatment to be extremely beneficial forms of bodywork. You can learn and practice these disciplines after you have your basic massage license (if required by your state). You can also go into research and/or writing on massage topics. There is a great need for scholarship in the massage field (just be careful not to develop carpal tunnel syndrome from too much computer typing!).

Think also about your lifestyle. Do you have another passion in life that requires you to use your hands intensively? If you love playing the piano two hours each day, or you need to do computer work to supplement your income, or you enjoy doing carpentry or gardening and do it regularly, you should think twice about becoming a full-time massage therapist. Doing two hand-intensive activities substantially increases your chances of becoming injured.

Being realistic about your strengths and weaknesses, and about what it takes to be a massage therapist, will give you a much better chance of staying healthy as you work in the profession. It may also give you the flexibility to consider some options you had not thought of before. Either way, it will help you save your hands.

2

Why Do Massage Therapists Get Injured?

Injury happens when the body is stressed beyond its own limits. Massage-related injury is caused by three main factors: the physical work of doing massage; predisposing characteristics of the massage therapist's body; and unhealthy work situations and expectations. This chapter examines each of these factors and how they add up to cause injury.

The Physical Work of Doing Massage

Repetitive Motion

Repetitive motion is the primary reason that massage causes injury. No one part of the body is designed to do the same motion over and over for long periods of time without rest. Each body part, depending on its size and strength, has its own limit as to how many times it can move in a certain way before the movement becomes too strenuous and tissue damage starts to occur. Take, for example, a technique commonly called "alternating thumbs," which requires the therapist to move both thumbs alternately in small circles at the

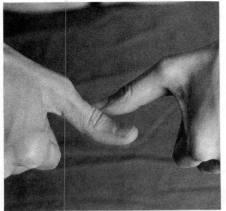

Photo 1

same time (Photo 1). Try making this motion in the air in front of you. You will probably notice that your thumbs start to get tired after just 15 or 20 circles. After 50, 75, or 100 circles, you will feel even more tired. How tired the thumbs get will vary from person to person, depending on their strength and other factors. The muscles in the thumb are quite small, and are not built to withstand repetitive demands on their limited strength.

Using Pressure and/or Weight

Do the "alternating thumbs" motion again, but this time do it on your thigh, pressing into the muscle as you repetitively move your thumbs. You have considerably increased the possibility of stressing your thumbs beyond their limits. Doing the same repetitive motion will take more strength now that you are using pressure produced by your muscle strength and/or your body weight. In addition, you are now putting stress on your entire upper extremity, not just your thumbs.

Stressful or Awkward Positioning of the Body

The human body is designed to distribute stress most efficiently when joints are lined up in a neutral position. No joint is flexed, extended, abducted, or adducted. In a neutral position, the joints and the muscles can create motion with the least possible amount of stress to the musculoskeletal system. Neutral positioning gives you a biomechanical advantage. Joints and muscles from adjacent structures work together to create movement instead of one isolated area doing all the work. For example, when you bend from the waist to pick up a heavy object, the flexion forces you to use your back alone to lift the weight. The act of lifting puts extra stress on the low back where flexion occurs. If you had kept your back straight, you would have been able to use the strong muscles of the hips and the legs to help you lift the weight.

Some stress to the body is unavoidable just from everyday living; after all, we spend very little time each day in a neutral position. After many years of normal, day-to-day stress, the joints do wear, and degenerative joint disease (DJD) sets in. Excessive amounts of stress can accelerate that process, or cause other kinds of injury.

To illustrate the effect of stressful or awkward positioning, move your muscles and joints out of alignment as you continue the repetitive "alternating thumbs" motion with pressure (Photo 2). With your hands and arms out of alignment, the muscles and joints have to work harder to accomplish the desired effect. By taking your upper limbs away from the midline toward the right side, you also have created greater stress to the right side of the body instead of distributing stress evenly to both sides. You might not believe anyone would work like this, but the author has seen therapists working in positions as awkward as this one without being aware of it.

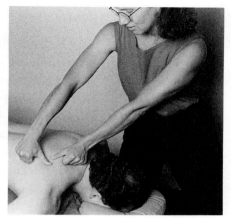

Photo 2

Generally, doing massage involves a combination of repetitive motion and pressure. When stressful or awkward positioning is added into the equation, the chances of injury as a result of doing massage increase. If an activity is repetitive enough, it does not even take a great deal of pressure, or extreme positioning, to cause injury. We hear so much these days about computer operators who develop carpal tunnel syndrome (see Chapter 4). The motion involved in typing on a computer keyboard is very small and subtle, involving flexion of the fingers. However, doing this motion thousands of times each day can cause injury. Hitting the keys too hard, or typing with the wrists out of neutral position, can turn the seemingly innocuous activity of typing into one of the leading causes of long-term occupation-related upper-extremity disability. The same combination of repetitiveness, pressure, and awkward positioning also makes doing massage potentially hazardous.

Predisposing Characteristics of the Massage Therapist

As we discussed previously, each person who does massage is different. Some bodies are better suited than others to withstand the stresses described above. Certain body characteristics can make a massage therapist more prone to injury. Developing awareness of the degree to which you have the following characteristics will help you protect yourself from being injured.

Lifestyle and General Health

These two factors play a significant role in the body's ability to withstand stress. A generally healthy, physically fit person is less likely to become injured from stressful activities than an unhealthy, deconditioned person. The healthy, fit person will also heal faster, so any small injury he sustains will resolve quickly rather than become more severe.

The amount of stress a body can take before injury occurs varies from individual to individual, depending on a number of factors (Table 1). One person can lift a 25 lb. weight with a flexed spine and be fine, while another might do the same and injure his back.

TABLE 1

Factors that play a role in your ability to
withstand mechanical stress

Age	Diet
Overall health (physical and mental)	Quality of circulation
Strength of muscles and bones	Aerobic fitness level
Diseases of the musculoskeletal system	Joint stability
Previous injuries	Stress level
Lifestyle (sleep, exercise, work habits)	Use of alcohol, drugs, or tobacco

---

The state of your health and the way you live day to day affect your ability to withstand the demands of a massage career. Factors such as smoking, poor nutrition (diet), lack of sleep, any past or present disease (either systemic or local), depression, and stress all have a negative impact on your body's function and ability to heal. Age also factors into the equation. All else being equal, a 45 year-old person heals more slowly than a 25 year-old person.

If you have had previous injuries, especially to the head, neck, spine, or upper extremity, you will be more prone to developing massage-related upper extremity injury. Motor vehicle accidents can be especially problematic, since they often cause soft tissue and nerve damage that is slow to resolve. You may not have any symptoms at this time, but the injury may still exist subclinically to some degree. Even after you heal, a previous injury can leave you with scarring or post-traumatic arthritis that can affect your ability to withstand additional stress to the area. The physical work of doing massage may aggravate the injury site, bringing back the original symptoms or creating new ones. The injury also may have caused some weakness in a joint or muscle that will cause you trouble in your massage work. One of the students in my workshops had broken one of her wrists, and had a history of carpal tunnel syndrome in both wrists. With these injuries in her past, she is at high risk of developing a massage-related injury.

Is there any hope for the out-of-shape, weak massage therapist? Of course. Again, the best defense against injury is developing body awareness. Be honest with yourself, and adapt to your strengths and weaknesses. If you are in poor condition, get into an exercise program (see your doctor first). If you have an unhealthy lifestyle, start making changes to improve it. If you have previous injuries, be on the lookout for signs of unresolved inflammation or weakness and treat them promptly. If you have many limitations and you aren't certain that they can all be overcome, think about doing a kind of massage that calls for less strength and endurance. The factors mentioned above make the massage therapist *prone* to injury. They do *not* make injury a foregone conclusion.

Conditioning and Circulation

The body needs a certain amount of regular activity to maintain good circulation, endurance and strength. We call someone who does not maintain this healthy level of activity "out-of-shape" or "deconditioned." People who are out of shape are usually inactive, lead sedentary lives, don't work out very much, tend to take the elevator instead of the stairs, or drive the car instead of walking. This inactivity eventually leads to poor circulation. Certain systemic disorders or diseases, such as heart disease and diabetes, can also impair circulation. Good circulation is necessary to the body's healing process. When tissue is damaged, blood flows into the injured area to bring in necessary nutrients and sweep away dead cells and waste products that impede healing. An injury sustained by a massage therapist who is in good shape and has good circulation will therefore heal faster and better than one sustained by a therapist who is out of shape or has a disorder that causes poor circulation.

Lack of circulation in muscles and tendons make these tissues rigid, less flexible and less resilient. Rigid tissues tear more easily than flexible ones, just as a tree that does not bend in the wind is more likely to break. For this reason, athletes are always cautioned to "warm up" their muscles before putting any strain on them. Gentle activity gets the blood flowing into the tissues, making them pliable, ready to work, and less likely to tear.

Like any athlete, the massage therapist needs to attain a basic level of muscular and cardiovascular conditioning before attempting to do massage work that requires strength and endurance (as almost all mainstream massage work does). A runner would not attempt a 10K race if she could not run more than 2K without gasping for breath and getting leg cramps. Neither should a massage therapist expect to give a one-hour, deep tissue massage if she can't do a few sit-ups and push-ups without getting tired, nor run around the block without getting winded.

Size of Muscles, Bones and Joints (Body Type)

A small build is a disadvantage for doing massage. The smaller and more delicate the muscles, bones and joints are, the more easily they can be damaged. It will take less stress to injure the small bones and joints of a delicately built person than to injure a person with a larger, more sturdy frame. If your build is small and/or delicate, you will have to compensate in other ways for the lack of pure physical heft that bigger people can bring to their work. You may need to use techniques in your work that put less emphasis on muscle and joint strength. You can also maximize your muscle power by getting into a strengthening exercise program like the one in Chapter 7.

Having a large build does not necessarily mean you will not get injured. As discussed in this chapter, you may have other body characteristics that can make you vulnerable to injury.

Strength

Most massage therapists perform tasks in their massages that require strength. If you possess less than the required strength to perform a particular task, you are likely to become injured from doing that task. For example: you are asked to lift a 200 pound weight over your head. You have never been able to lift even a fifty pound weight over your head in the past, so you know you do not have the necessary strength to accomplish this task. If you force yourself to lift the 200 pound weight anyway, you will stress your body beyond its own limits, and the result will be an injury. Certainly, you will not be lifting 200 pound weights as a massage therapist. However, you may lift a client's head (14-15 pounds average) and hold it raised for five minutes as you massage the back of the neck, or you may lift his leg (anywhere from 15 to 100 pounds) to do range of motion testing at the hip. Do you have the strength to lift these body parts?

We tend not to think about how much a body part weighs before we lift it. You would think twice about lifting a box of books marked 100 pounds, but a leg weighing the same amount appears to be just a mass of tissue that needs massaging. Even when the therapist's hand or arm starts to shake from the strain of this lifting, she will often disregard this indication of insufficient strength and excessive stress and deem it a necessary aspect of delivering the treatment. The author has seen a number of massage therapists who look like they could not lift a 20 pound weight nonchalantly lifting a shoulder or a leg of a muscular man, and straining with the effort.

Lifting is not the only massage maneuver that requires strength. When you use your own body weight to apply pressure to a client's tissues, your upper extremity has to support that weight. Do you have the upper body strength to support one-third to one-half of your own weight? Remember also that weak muscles still may be able to respond to over-stressful tasks in a short burst. They will tire very quickly, though, and start performing less and less well. In a short span of time, they can tear from the stress.

Joint Instability — Too Much of a Good Thing

Good ROM is usually a desirable quality because it allows the greatest freedom of movement. When ROM is greater than normal, the bones and muscles that connect at the joint can be put under excessive stress.

Some persons are born with loose joints: it is a hereditary characteristic. One place where a loose joint may be particularly problematic is at the base of the thumb. Perhaps you are one of those people who has always been able to bend the thumb backward until it creates a 90 degree angle with the rest of the hand. If so, you have greater than normal ROM in your thumb. The ligaments that hold the

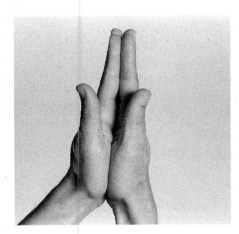

Photo 3

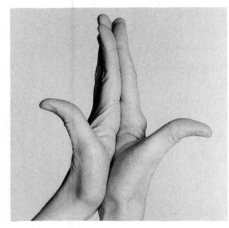

Photo 4

thumb in place and limit its range of motion are looser and less restrictive than in most other people. The thumb is congenitally hypermobile, or excessively movable. If your thumb became hypermobile sometime after birth, it may have been the result of an injury, for example from a fall or a blow. In that case, you may have sprained the ligaments in the thumb, which means you partially or totally tore them. Without the support of strong, protectively restricting ligaments, the thumb becomes hypermobile.

Hypermobile joints get out of alignment more easily. The therapist with overly flexible joints is more likely to get into awkward or stressful positions when giving massage. If the therapist puts pressure on the unstable thumb joint in his massage work, the thumb starts to wobble. It will require more concentration and muscular control to steady the thumb. The extra work the muscles have to do to hold the thumb steady can overstress them and cause tissue damage. Any time the therapist becomes distracted and loses concentration, the muscular control will decrease, and the thumb will start to wobble again. When he places pressure on the thumb, it will naturally fall into a stressful or awkward position, creating stress to the joint that can result in injury.

A good way to start developing awareness of how well your body is adapted to doing massage is to examine the stability of your joints. Start by looking again at the ROM of the carpometacarpal joint at the base of the thumbs, also known as the saddle joint. Put your palms together in front of you ("prayer" position) and extend your thumbs laterally, away from the midline of the body (Photo 3). Be sure you are extending your thumbs out to the sides, not abducting them toward your body. If you feel any pain or discomfort, back off a bit. How far do your thumbs go out to the sides? A small amount (Photo 3), quite a bit (Photo 4), or somewhere between the two? What about ROM at the interphalangeal joint of the thumb? Does the distal phalangeal bone stay upright over the joint, or does the end of the thumb bend backward away from the joint (Photo 5)?

Thumbs tend to be hypermobile in part by virtue of their structure. The carpometacarpal joint, the only saddle joint in the body, allows increased ROM to make the thumb opposable. This extra ROM allows us to grasp objects in our hands. This naturally large ROM makes it more difficult to hold the thumb in alignment. Any additional ROM caused by congenital hypermobility or ligament sprain will make the thumb even more prone to injury. You can begin to see why massage therapists so often injure their thumbs.

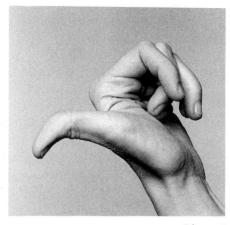

Photo 5

If you have an appropriate ROM in your thumbs, you will be better able to keep them straight and stable when you use them in your massage routines. If you have excessive ROM in your thumbs, make a mental note of this limitation and remain aware of it in your work. You should limit the use of your thumbs in massage. In fact, because of the thumb's inherent hypermobility, all massage therapists should be careful not to overuse their thumbs in their work. See Chapter 6 for further discussion of proper thumb use.

Another important place to look for possible instability is at the wrist. Put your hands up in front of you with your forearms flexed at the elbow and your palms facing away from your body, like a traffic cop saying "Stop". You are going to isolate movement at the wrist, so be sure to keep your forearms absolutely straight up and down as you move your hands. Take your wrists only as far as they will comfortably go. If you feel any pain or discomfort, back off a bit. First, move your hands into radial deviation at the wrist (Photo 6). Do you have a little range of motion in radial deviation at the wrists (Photo 6), excessive motion (Photo 7), or somewhere between the two?

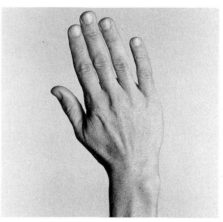

Photo 6

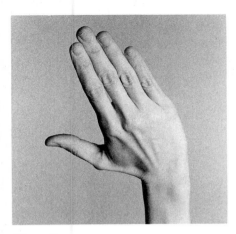

Photo 7

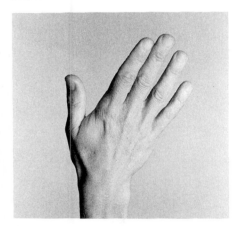

Photo 8

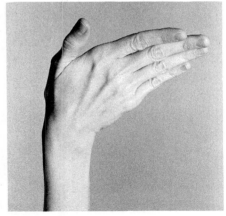

Photo 9

Return the hands to neutral. Now take your hands into ulnar deviation by moving the hands laterally, or away from the midline (Photo 8). Once again, make sure you keep your forearms straight up and down. Ask yourself the same question: do I have limited ROM in ulnar deviation (Photo 8), greater than normal ROM (Photo 9), or somewhere between the two?

Sometimes joint instability can amplify repetitive motion. For example, ligament damage between the carpal bones can exacerbate any larger repetitive motion happening at the wrist. If there is a repetitive movement of ulnar deviation at the wrist, the carpal bones at the ulnar side of the hand will move around each other as the hand moves. A smaller repetitive movement is created within the larger repetitive motion of ulnar deviation at the wrist. Either one of these repetitive movements can cause an injury at the wrist; the two together can make injury happen faster, or increase its severity.

Just to be clear: Doing massage does not cause ligament tears (sprain). Ligaments are made up of strong, fibrous connective tissue that only breaks or tears with trauma, such as a hard sudden blow or a fall. Massage, although stressful in other ways, is usually not stressful in a traumatic sense (unless you happen to slip on a drop of oil and fall on your client!). However, doing massage improperly or excessively can cause ligaments to stretch slightly. As we discussed above, lax ligaments can create joint instability and the problems associated with it.

Remember that even a very strong, broadly-built person who is in very good shape and has no predisposing characteristics will eventually hit her limit. Surpassing that limit will overtax her body and cause injury. It is often external or emotional forces that push a person who is otherwise well-suited to doing massage over the limit. Some of these are described below.

Unhealthy Work Situations and Expectations

It would be wonderful if we could all do massage under the best possible conditions at all times. As those who have been massage therapists for a while know, this is more often the exception than the rule. Sometimes the conditions under which you have to work will be less than ideal. However, if you are aware of the potential dangers of these situations, you will be able to make an effort to control your work conditions as much as possible so you can stay healthy.

Suddenly Increasing the Number of Massages You Do

Like any athlete, a massage therapist must *train* in order to become physically capable of taking on increased amounts of physical activity. Let's go back to our runner example, the one who is currently able to comfortably run two kilometers per day before her body starts showing signs of giving out under the stress. If her eventual goal is to be able to run a 10K race without getting injured, she must start a training program to develop sufficient strength and endurance to meet that goal. She will slowly increase the length and intensity of her daily runs, monitoring her body (pulse rate, respiration rate, muscle aching or weakening) to make sure it is handling the added stress. With a slow, steady increase in activity, she will allow her body to adapt to the increased demands placed on it while remaining healthy.

The massage therapist who wants to increase the number of massages he does each day or each week must adopt the model of the athlete in training. A gradual increase in physically demanding activity slowly and steadily builds strength and endurance without injury. Any sudden increase in massage activity, such as doing two massages one week and six massages the next week, increases the risk of being injured.

Suddenly Decreasing the Time You Take Between Massages

Decreasing the amount of time you take between massages also will make you more prone to injury. The body needs time to rest between periods of physical exertion. The runner we mentioned above would certainly not go out and run another 10K race only an hour after the first one! Neither should the massage therapist do two massages in a row with only enough time between them to change the sheets. The more time you can leave between massages, the more time your body will have to rest and heal, which will help you prevent injury.

Regulating massage workload is an issue for both the student and the professional. Students generally are required to do several massages per week for school, and may do several more for friends and family to practice techniques. If a student volunteers at a local sports event in addition to her schoolwork, she may be asked to do five to ten massages on the day of the event. Since she has never done more than one or two massages in one day previously, she may end up with the beginnings of an injury by the end of the day.

The student who has just graduated from school and become licensed also has a challenge ahead of him. He probably is anxious to begin his practice, and impatient to have as many clients as possible as soon as possible. If he gives in to these tendencies and immediately acquires a full workload, he may become injured.

The professional massage therapist may find that her workload varies greatly from week to week, or month to month. She may give ten massages one week, then have a slow week with only three massages, and then have a holiday spurt where everyone who ever got a gift certificate for her services wants a massage in the same week. She does not want to say no to all these new customers, so she gives twenty or twenty-five massages that week. This kind of schedule can cause injury. An aware therapist who attempts to balance economic considerations with the potential for injury is more likely to have a long and healthy career.

Massaging in Pressured Situations

Imagine this scenario. It is your first week working for a clinic on their massage staff. Your boss is very demanding, and you know you need to make a good impression on her to keep this job. After the fourth massage of the morning, your hands start to hurt. You try not to think about it -- maybe it'll go away. So you ignore the pain that first day, and the next, and the next after that. You do a great job, and the boss loves you, but now you are in pain every day and it is getting worse. What do you do now?

Giving massage under this kind of pressure to perforrm, whether it is external or self-imposed, will put you in a precarious situation. You are too uptight to pay attention to anything that may interfere with your performance, including the signals your body is sending you that it is overstressed. If you are a student, you may feel that to get a good grade you have to show your instructor that you have no problem at all with a technique that makes your wrists hurt. If you are working professionally, your body mechanics may go out the window because you are too preoccupied with giving your client the best treatment of his life so he will tell your supervisor how great you are. Perhaps your toughest critic is yourself, and it is your own excessively high standards that must be met at all costs. Whatever the source of the pressure, it has the same result: it overpowers your awareness and your ability to change your behavior to protect yourself from injury.

Working under pressure like this can cause your muscles to become overly tense. If your muscles are already contracted from emotional tension, they will not be able to rest between tasks. When the already overburdened muscles have to do massage work, the additional contraction you ask of them may be more than they can withstand. They will be more likely to tear in this situation and become injured.

Try to avoid pressured situations as much as possible. For those that cannot be avoided, make a plan of action for yourself that will allow you to maintain your body awareness while you work. For tips on staying healthy while dealing with work and school pressures, see Chapter 9.

Massaging In a Cramped Room

Without sufficient space in your massage room, you will be likely to get into awkward or stressful positions as you massage. For example, if you are forced to stand at the side of the table to work on the feet (because there isn't enough room for you to stand at the end of the table), you may find yourself bending your upper body and hands to the side as you attempt to address the length of the foot (see photo 41, Chapter 6). This position would put stress not only on your upper extremity, but also on your back, and could lead to injury if done often enough. To work most efficiently, you need enough room around the table so that you can stand in whatever place is most comfortable for any given technique. If you are comfortable, your body will be more likely to assume relaxed, efficient, naturally aligned postures while you are massaging.

Arrange your massage space to create as much space as possible around the table. If you are stuck working in a cramped room, monitor yourself carefully to avoid unhealthy positioning and distorted body mechanics.

Massaging With Your Table at an Uncomfortable Height

Table height is a popular subject of debate among massage therapists. Some insist that one needs leverage to promote good body mechanics, and that means the table must be relatively low. Others maintain that the table should be at a higher level so the therapist doesn't have to be reaching down to the client or bending over her.

Finding a table height that allows you to maintain good body positioning as you massage is extremely important. However, there is no right or wrong table height per se. Table height is really a matter of personal preference and comfort. As you develop greater body awareness, you will be more sensitive to which table height works best for you at any given moment. The problem is that a stationary table may be the right height for working on one client, and the wrong height for working on another. A 200 pound person may add six inches to the height of your table when he lies down on it, while a slight person may add only three inches. The height of some tables can be adjusted by shortening or lengthening the legs manually between clients, which is helpful up to a point. However, most massage therapists (and physical therapists, too) find that they need to change table height several times during a massage to accommodate different techniques. Some therapists use a step stool if they need to raise themselves above the client for certain techniques. These should be used with great care, since they can be quite unstable and cause you to be off-balance as you work.

An ideal solution is to invest in a hydraulic or electric table. These tables give you a full range of heights from which to choose at any time, just by flicking a switch or stepping on a foot pedal. You can change the table height every time you change technique or area of the body, if you wish, and the client will remain undisturbed. At the time of this printing, a good stationary, adjustable massage table costs between $499 and $699. A good, basic hydraulic or electric massage table runs between $1999 and $2199. Although the price of a hydraulic table is considerably higher than a regular table, the comfort and possible injury protection it offers make it an investment worth considering.

Massaging When You Are Tired

Physical performance begins to suffer when fatigue starts to set in. Your strength may no longer be sufficient to perform the tasks at hand. Fatigue also will erode your attention to proper positioning and technique. When you are tired, you do not react as quickly to stimuli, including pain, that may be signalling you to stop or change what you are doing. It is important to learn to recognize the point at which fatigue starts affecting your massage work. Continuing to massage beyond that point can set the stage for injury to occur.

Doing Other Hand-Intensive Activities

There are many vocations and avocations that involve rigorous use of the hands and arms. Playing an instrument, typing on a computer, building furniture, and gardening are all hand-intensive activities. Doing activities like these in addition to giving massages may well be too much for your hands and arms to take. The more you use your hands, the more likely you are to injure them. The author once received a phone call from a massage therapist who gave massages part-time, did computer work part-time, and also played the piano several hours each day. She wondered why her hands were starting to hurt all the time. The answer was obvious: she was simply asking too much of her hands, and they were starting to rebel and tell her to cut it out! To stay healthy as a massage therapist, you will need to cut down on the amount of other work you ask your upper extremities to do. A part-time career as a professional solo violinist, in addition to your massage work, is probably not a healthy idea.

Believing in "No Pain, No Gain"

Massage therapists have traditionally suffered silently with pain and injury. Some therapists are convinced that this suffering comes with the profession and must simply be tolerated. They may have a hard time understanding why you are "making such a big deal" about being in pain. They may even be proud of their pain, and look down on those who complain as "wimps" or "amateurs." This unhealthy attitude gets passed on to their clients ("don't worry -- it's no big deal") and their students if they teach massage.

Sports medicine has taught us in recent years that the "no pain, no gain" attitude is counterproductive. Pain does not have to be a by-product of physical activity; in fact, it is to be avoided. Pain cannot be overcome by being "tough" or "not giving in to it." A smart therapist figures out why he is in pain and makes the changes necessary to get rid of it. One can only wonder how many of those therapists who learned to live with pain ended up having to stop massaging because of injury!

Feeling It Is Shameful to Be Injured

Since massage is all about health and well-being, it seems incongruous for the person doing massage to be anything less than in perfect health. Massage therapists want to feel that they can put themselves aside and pay attention only to the client. They do not talk much about injury, and when they do it is with fear and shame. Students feel particularly ashamed to say they are injured, that they cannot keep up with their classmates who seem able to concentrate only on learning techniques and helping their clients. Therapists who can ignore their problems get positive feedback, and therapists who cannot get very little support.

These unrealistic expectations only serve to make it more likely that massage therapists will be injured. Many therapists try to ignore their symptoms, hoping that they will go away by themselves (they usually do not). Others say the pain is not bad, that they can massage through it. They rationalize that they have not really been doing much massage, when they are still doing as many massages as ever. They put off treatment, saying they just need to get through the next quarter at school or the next week full of clients, then they will take a rest.

Do not take chances with your career and your health. There is nothing shameful about getting injured: it happens to massage therapists all the time. If you have pain while you do massage, you need to address why it is happening and correct the problem. If you are beginning to find everyday activities like tying your shoes and brushing your teeth to be painful, you are definitely having a problem. You wouldn't let a client ignore their symptoms of injury. Don't you deserve the same consideration?

Listen to and trust your instincts. Unless you are an alarmist, that little voice in your head that says "something is just not right" is telling you something important. With increased body awareness, that voice can become quite adept at determining whether you are injured.

Remember, though, that symptoms can be very confusing, and no one expects you to be able to diagnose yourself. If it is unclear to you whether you are injured or not, see a health professional who is trained to treat this type of injury. It is much better to err on the side of caution than to allow an injury to go untreated.

Believing There Is a "Right" and "Wrong" Way to Do Massage

Students and new graduates often feel they must incorporate every technique they were ever taught in school into their massages, even those techniques that they find uncomfortable or painful. They think the way they were taught to massage in school is the "right" way to do massage, and that massaging any other way is "wrong." This inflexibility puts pressure on you and keeps you from finding the way of doing massage that is best adapted to your own body's strengths and limitations. In other words, it closes the door on the body awareness that could keep you from being injured. It also stifles your creativity, which is a shame.

Massage is an art. There is no one right way of doing it. What you learn in school is a good basis from which to develop your own style. Once you are a professional, you can experiment and find the massage techniques you like best, adapt others to your own body's characteristics, and after a while, abandon the ones that don't feel like "you." Most importantly, you can stop doing the ones that hurt. Follow this simple axiom: *if it hurts, don't do it.* Give yourself permission take care of yourself, to say "no" to anything that may cause you to be injured.

The Myth of the "Good" Massage

Another misconception is that there is one definition of what constitutes a "good" massage and a "bad" massage. Many massage therapists feel that a "good" massage is one in which most of the time is spent working on small areas using a great deal of pressure. "More is better" is their motto. If a little treatment is good, a lot of treatment is better. If some pressure affects the muscles, a lot of pressure will really make them respond. A "good" massage, for these practitioners, is one in which they exhaust themselves (and likely their clients as well) and put their hands and arms under tremendous stress.

There is no standard for what constitutes a "good" massage. Each client will have his own opinion on the subject, depending on his own tastes and physical condition. Certainly, a client with an acute injury and fibromyalgia will not respond well to forty-five minutes of painful trigger point work in one area followed by tapotement, even if the therapist is convinced that every massage must contain those techniques. The more flexible you become about your own work, the more open you will be to the client's real needs, and the better able you will be to respond appropriately.

A massage therapist related an experience she had with a client that completely changed her ideas about what made a "good" massage. The client was a seventy-five year-old man who was referred to her by his physician with a diagnosis of insomnia. The therapist started the massage with her usual array of moves, and within five minutes, the client had fallen into a deep sleep. She was not quite sure what to do next. If she had continued to go through her regular routine, she would certainly have woken him up. Following her instincts, she sat down in a chair next to the table, laid her hand on his back, and stroked him very gently. Close to the end of the session, he woke up. He was very happy with the treatment, and wanted to come back and see her again for another session. He had achieved his goal in seeking massage treatment: he was able to sleep. The therapist felt that this massage was one of the best she had ever given.

As you develop the flexibility to accept your unique body characteristics and massage style, you will become more receptive to the wide range of body types and conditions that you will see in your clients. Like you, each client is unique and needs to be treated as an individual. Each massage session with that client will be unique and different from the last one. Working *with* your clients' unique characteristics and your own instead of against them will not only keep you healthy, but will make your work richer, more varied, and more rewarding.

3

Understanding the Injury Process

To have a clear understanding of why injury happens to massage therapists, you need to understand the physiology of injury, in other words, how the body responds to excessive physical stress on a cellular level. Understanding the extent to which stress can change and damage your tissues can encourage you to listen more attentively to any symptoms you may develop, and to seek appropriate treatment more swiftly. Students may find this section covers completely new material, facts they need to know to help them prevent injury. Professionals can benefit from this information as a review of principles they need to know to protect their own health and to treat their clients. This chapter also offers a concise, clear way to explain the injury process to clients.

Injury Physiology

We said earlier that injury happens when the body is stressed beyond its limits. We also examined how strenuous massage can cause this kind of stress. The overloading or overstressing of tissues as a result of doing massage occurs when:

1. Muscle/tendon tissue is overstretched;
2. Muscle/tendon tissue is overshortened from repetitive muscular contraction; and/or
3. Tendons, tendon sheaths, or nerves are impinged.
4. Joints are overloaded by repetitive use.

An injury may occur as a result of one or more of these four factors occurring at the same time. Any of the first three can create trauma and subsequent damage to the muscle/tendon fibers in the form of small rips, or microtears. Overstretching can also cause large tears, or macrotears, but this degree of damage is associated more with violent or sudden trauma than it is with the kind of gradual overstressing of tissues involved in doing massage.

Microtearing in itself does not necessarily lead to injury. In fact, it is a normal part of the wear and tear the musculoskeletal system undergoes every day. What, then, makes the difference between microtearing that doesn't lead to injury, and microtearing that does lead to injury? The key is healing time. Body builders, for example, are instructed to take a day off between weight-lifting sessions to give their muscles time to rest and heal before they put stress on them again. Repetition of trauma without adequate healing time has a cumulative effect on the muscles and tendons. Adequate healing time will vary from individual to individual. Furthermore, as the trauma continues unabated, the injury becomes more and more severe.

The body responds to injury on several levels. On the most basic level, micro- and macrotearing damages or kills the cells that make up the muscle/tendon. As the cell membrane loses its integrity, the contents of the cell spill out into the surrounding tissue. The contents include chemical mediators that trigger the body's inflammatory response. Acute inflammation is the reaction of the tissues to local injury. It involves a series of changes that occur as the body begins to repair itself and replace damaged or dead tissue with healthy tissue.

Tissue repair begins early in the inflammatory process. Muscle and tendon cells are permanent cells that, once dead, cannot regenerate. Instead, the body replaces the original tissue with connective tissue patches, in the process we know as scarring. Scar tissue serves to reattach the portions of tissue that have been torn. New scar tissue is weak; with time and relief from the trauma that caused the injury, the scar tissue heals and becomes a structural part of the muscle or tendon. However, if there is additional trauma to the injury site while the scar tissue is still immature and weak, it can be reinjured easily. The scar tissue breaks, inflammation sets in, and the process of tissue replacement begins again. The longer the trauma goes on without adequate healing time, the more scar tissue is produced at the injury site.

This process can progress past the point where enough scar tissue has been created to adequately repair the tear. Given the nature of muscle and tendon tissue, this overabundance of scar tissue can cause as many problems as it was originally supposed to fix. Muscles and tendons are made up of fibers that run parallel to each other. This formation allows them to slide smoothly over each other as the muscle or tendon contracts. Scar tissue tends to form unevenly, with collagen fibers crisscrossing each other in every direction, forming a messy patch of fibers lying on top of each other. Massage or gentle mobilization can help straighten out these fibers. If the injured area is immobilized or left untreated, the scar tissue causes the muscle fibers to adhere to each other, binding them together so they are no longer lying parallel to each other. Scar tissue also can tack the muscle to other structures in the area, such as bone. As the scar tissue matures, it hardens, stiffens and contracts, forming hard masses or adhesions at the points where the fibers have stuck together. Where the adhesions form, the fibers can no longer glide smoothly over each other, but rather rub against each other, creating friction that causes more inflammation. If hard, stiff scar tissue forms near or at a joint, it can interfere with the movement of the bones at that joint. Adhesions and scar tissue masses are the objects of a good deal of your work as a massage therapist. Those hard, crunchy spots you find in your clients are sites of past injury and inflammation from overuse or other trauma. Massage can be quite effective at breaking up young scar tissue to restore movement and relieve pain.

The injury/reinjury cycle often operates in the kind of injuries sustained by massage therapists. If you create micro- or macrotears in muscle or tendon tissue in your upper extremity from doing massage, your body will react to this injury by producing inflammation. Given enough time and rest, the inflammation will dissipate, an appropriate amount of scar tissue will form, and the area will heal properly. However, if you re-traumatize the affected area by continuing to do the same thing that got you injured in the first place, you will cause more inflammation, followed by more scarring. This process will continue as long as the trauma continues. As more and more scar tissue builds up at the injury site, you may begin to develop adhesions and other masses of scar tissue that can cause pain, more inflammation, and limitation of function, starting the cycle all over again.

If the injury is at a joint, another type of cycle can be set in motion as well. Inflammation or scar tissue in the joint cavity can change the synovial fluid. The synovial fluid thins out and become less viscous, so it provides less cushioning to the bones of the joint. Without that cushioning, the cartilage at the joint surfaces will begin to degenerate, making the joint space smaller and reducing the cushion between the bones. Inflammation in itself can also damage the cartilage. Subsequent wear on the bones causes bone spurs to appear. We recognize these changes as osteoarthritis or degenerative joint disease (DJD).

Symptoms of Injury

When inflammation has progressed to a sufficient level to trigger pain receptors, your body starts sending you signals that something bad is happening. Your challenge is to learn to recognize these signals, or symptoms, as warning signs that something is wrong. Learning to listen to your body is a crucial step in developing the important body awareness that will enable you to protect yourself and stay healthy as you do massage. The ability to recognize the very first mild symptoms of injury is extremely important. By the time you are able to perceive symptoms, degenerative changes may have already started taking place in your tissues. The longer the injury remains untreated, the more difficult it will be to resolve. Catching the injury early will help you keep your tissues healthy, preventing the vicious cycles of inflammation, injury and reinjury.

There are five cardinal signs of an inflammatory process. An easy way to remember them is with the acronym **SH(a)RP-L**:

Swelling (edema)

Heat

("a" is there just to make the word)

Redness

Pain

Loss of Function

One, several, or all of these signs may be present at any one time. In addition to these signs of inflammation, you may experience other symptoms associated with injury (Table 2). Any of these symptoms, alone or in combination, can be an indication that tissue damage has occurred.

Table 2

Additional Upper Extremity Symptoms Associated With Injury

Feeling of heaviness
Fatigue
Tightness (muscle hypertonicity)
Hypersensitivity (e.g., wearing a watch or being touched on the affected on the affected limb is intolerable)
Everyday activities reproduce your pain (e.g., opening a jar, doorknob, car window or faucet, brushing your hair or teeth, or writing)
Achiness
Burning
Crepitation (popping or clicking when joints move)
Twinges
Numbness and tingling (paresthesias)
Involuntary or uncoordinated movements such as tremors, twitches, tics, sudden flexion/extension of fingers, inability to hold objects steady in hand
Clumsiness
Hesitation to use the "bad" arm or hand to hold objects or support your weight
The realization that your hands have not felt "normal" for a while, like they did before you started doing massage

---

The primary and most common warning sign of injury is pain. Pain that does not resolve quickly is *always* a sign that something is wrong. The word "pain" can be a very subjective term that is used differently by different people. You may say you feel "pain" after a good workout, and wake up fine and healthy the next morning. You may also say you feel "pain" after you have run a marathon, and wake up the next morning with a swollen, injured knee.

It is important to be able to differentiate between the sensations associated with normal use of the body and those associated with injury. We can assign some general characteristics to "pain" associated with normal use and "pain" associated with injury to help us determine when we have crossed the line between the two (Table 3). Each person will draw that line in a different place. With increased understanding and awareness of your body, you will start to get a sense of the point at which your pain enters the realm of injury. This awareness will help you evaluate the symptoms you are experiencing and decide whether you just need to rest, adjust your activity, or seek treatment for an injury.

Table 3

Features of Pain Associated With Normal Use vs.
Pain Expected From Injury

	Normal Use	From Injury
Severity	mild to moderate	tends to be more severe
Character	more dull than sharp, achy, sore	usually sharper
Location	diffuse, generalized	tends to be localized
Affected Areas	usually bilateral	usually unilateral
Duration	lessens & disappears in 24-48 hrs.	persists after 48 hrs., either constantly or recurrently
Associated Symptoms	some heat, muscle stiffness and tightness only	SH(A)RP-L, paresthesias, etc.

Remember that these are very general parameters. The only features listed above that always indicate injury are swelling, redness, loss of function (not to be confused with mild stiffness) and persistence over time. Rather than provide you with an exact scale by which to measure what is pain from use and what is injury pain, the pain's *characteristics* should stimulate reflection when you have symptoms after activity. After a long day of massage, when your hands and/or arms don't feel quite right, ask yourself: how severe is my pain? Is it more dull than sharp? After three days, are you still experiencing these symptoms? The answers to these questions will help you develop a profile of your condition, just like the answers your clients give you in their accounts of their symptoms.

Try to be as objective as you can in evaluating your symptoms. If you have a low pain threshold, you may categorize any pain as moderate to severe. You will need to develop a sense of proportion for what mild, moderate, and severe mean for you.

Many massage therapists hesitate to say they are "injured," preferring to think that it is normal to be in pain much of the time. In *Save Your Hands!* workshops, participants are asked to raise their hands if they are having any symptoms. Many of them raise their hands.

When those who raised their hands are asked if they feel they are "injured," very few say "yes." By the end of the workshop, they have usually changed their minds. They realize that they have been inappropriately minimizing the severity of their problems.

Even if you are certain you are not injured, pay attention to the signals your body is sending you. The reason you felt achiness, stiffness, or tightness is that you pushed the limits of what your body can do. You got a bit too close for comfort to that dividing line, and your body is letting you know it. You will need to rest and modify your activity before trying to do any more rigorous massage work, so you can avoid becoming injured.

4

Common Injuries Sustained by Massage Therapists

Now that you understand basic injury physiology and symptoms, you can apply this information to specific injuries. Each injury has its own set of characteristic or classic symptoms. This chapter will review common injury syndromes, including typical onset and etiology. This information will help you understand what is happening to you, and perhaps why it is happening, so you can start to make some informed decisions about modifying how you do massage, as well as how you choose treatment.

Soft tissue injuries common to massage therapists fall into two categories: muscle/tendon injuries and nerve impingement injuries. The primary cause of these disorders is thought to be overuse, or using a part of the body more than is considered normal or healthy. Left untreated or allowed to become chronic, these injuries can initiate the process of synovial thinning, and ultimately lead to post-traumatic osteoarthritis. They can also accelerate the natural process of joint degeneration and chronic osteoarthritis that occurs with aging.

You will often see injuries caused by overuse lumped together under the terms repetitive stress injuries (RSI's), cumulative trauma disorders (CTD's), or simply overuse syndromes. RSI's are often in the news these days, as public awareness grows about occupation-related upper extremity injury. Workers in professions that call for intense and/or repetitive use of their hands are prone to these injuries, including computer operators, hairstylists, carpenters, construction workers, assembly line workers, musicians, cashiers, and massage therapists.

Other health care workers sustain RSI's as well. In personal interviews, one physician's assistant in gynecology stated that she was developing a sore wrist from performing internal gynecological exams all day! Physical and occupational therapists report experiencing symptoms of injury from time to time as a result of the soft tissue work they do, including deep massage and myofascial release. In fact, several physical therapists expressed relief that they only had to do five or ten minutes of soft tissue work at a time with their clients; otherwise they would get injured as much as massage therapists do!

Repetitive stress injuries can be very confusing. They often overlap in causes and symptoms. You may start out with one kind of injury, and find that it develops into another kind of injury later on. Your symptoms may come and go, or be atypical and difficult to classify. In nerve impingement injuries, it can be difficult to determine the exact site of nerve compression, since symptoms can be felt at any point along the nerve pathway. It is also quite possible to have several problems at the same time, in which case you may have trouble distinguishing which problem is causing a particular symptom. New information comes out every day about these injuries, as the allopathic and alternative medical communities continue their research. The descriptions presented here reflect current accepted knowledge.

Muscle/Tendon Injuries

Overuse Syndrome

The commonly accepted definition of overuse syndrome is tissue damage caused by the cumulative effect of repetitively stressing the tissues beyond their anatomic and physiologic limits. Overuse syndrome is thought of as a chronic injury because of its gradual onset and generally long duration. There may be no definable "acute" stage to the injury, even though the symptoms may increase in severity at times. The most common injury sites in massage therapists are the thumb, the wrist, and the forearm, although overuse of the elbow and the shoulder also occur. The incidence of overuse syndrome seems to be higher in women than in men.

The medical literature contains much disagreement about the meaning and use of the terms "overuse syndrome" and "tendinitis/tenosynovitis," which are often used interchangeably to describe muscle/tendon injury. The reason for the confusion is the lack of reliable data to create adequately meaningful and concrete descriptions of each injury and define distinctions between the two. Medical science still does not completely understand what happens to the body in these injuries, nor exactly what causes them physiologically. However, in the past few years, researchers have begun to come to a consensus on the use of the term "overuse syndrome," which is now increasingly used to denote a condition with its own discrete etiology and symptoms independent and distinct from disorders like tendonitis/tenosynovitis.

We generally use the term "overuse syndrome" to mean a set of symptoms and physiologic changes that do not fit into any other specific syndrome of muscle/tendon injury. The symptoms and changes experienced by massage therapists most commonly fall into this category. Overuse syndrome is therefore the most common diagnosis given to injured massage therapists. The work we do involves subtle movements done repetitively for long periods (usually an hour or more at a time) without rest. This process slowly wears away at our upper extremities. Over time, little by little, tissue damage accumulates, and we begin to notice signs that something is wrong. This slow onset is one of the defining characteristics of this disorder.

The injury/reinjury cycle, described in Chapter 3, is the major contributing factor in overuse syndrome. You do some massage, your hands start to hurt, the tissues begin to be damaged, you ignore the pain and keep doing massage, reinjuring the tissues, causing more tissue damage, and the cycle repeats over and over again. The injury/reinjury cycle can be very hard to break, and makes overuse syndrome a difficult injury to treat. Injuries that have slow, complex causes tend to have slow resolutions.

It can take weeks, months or even years for overuse syndrome to develop. Onset occurs most often with a sudden and/or substantial increase in workload. A sudden decrease in time spent between massages can also precipitate the injury, as can changing technique or learning new techniques, or simply going through a period of psychological stress.

Degenerative changes at the joint surfaces and tendon sheaths begin a few weeks prior to the onset of the overuse disorder (the prodrome to the overuse syndrome). As the syndrome progresses, a number of physiological changes happen to the synovia and surrounding tissues. The muscles become contracted constantly, not allowing the tissues to relax and rest. As the overtired muscles become painful, they contract even more in response to the pain, creating a vicious cycle of pain-spasm-pain. Tendons become irritated at their attachments to bone and muscle. Synovial fluid thickens, and chemical changes happen in the fluids between the cells of the affected tissues. Ligaments can stretch from excessive use, causing pain and joint instability. Repetitive stress may cause microtearing of muscles and/or tendons, leading to inflammation and scar tissue formation, and contributes to an associated tendonitis. There is speculation that there is neurological involvement in the syndrome to some degree as well.

Symptoms can vary greatly from person to person afflicted with overuse syndrome. This is one of the reasons this injury is still not fully understood. The primary symptom associated with overuse syndrome is diffuse achiness, tightness and/or soreness in one part of the body rather than sharp pain in one location that can be pinpointed. This soreness can range from mild to severe. Twinges of pain may occur and may be quite severe, although short lived. Other symptoms that can appear in overuse syndrome include loss of function and the presence of paresthesias. Muscle bellies and tendons in the injured area may be tender to the touch. Crepitations, or crackling/ popping sounds, can often be heard in the injured tendons.

Classic signs of inflammation like swelling, redness and heat are generally not present in overuse syndrome. In fact, it has never been proven scientifically that inflammation is a clinical feature of overuse syndrome. In microscopic examination of tissue thought to be damaged in overuse syndrome, inflammation has not been found. Steroids and nonsteroidal anti-inflammatory medications have been found to be of limited efficacy in treating overuse syndrome, which supports the theory that inflammation is not part of the disorder.

In the early stages of the injury, pain may be mild to moderate and may be present only when the therapist is actually doing massage. Eventually, the severity of the pain increases and may also be present at rest and when using the upper extremity for other activities. Many therapists with advanced overuse syndrome experience pain while writing, brushing their hair, rolling down a car window, opening a jar, turning a faucet, or picking up a child. One therapist reported that the mere act of *reaching* to open a kitchen cabinet was excruciatingly painful for her. In the upper limb, overuse syndrome may begin in one arm and then spread to the other without any apparent cause.

Massage therapists suffering from overuse syndrome usually find that it takes quite a while for the injury to resolve completely. Some find that it goes away after a few months, or that it goes away at first and returns repeatedly over the course of a few years. Therapists have reported recovery periods ranging from one to five years.

In a typical overuse syndrome scenario, a massage therapist might begin slowly experiencing symptoms in the wrist of her dominant hand after a sudden increase in workload. The symptoms become more severe over time as she reinjures the area by continuing to do massage. The main symptom is pain, diffuse one day, more specific the next. There are no signs of inflammation: no redness, heat or swelling. At first, her wrist hurts only when she does massage. After a while, it hurts all the time, at rest and when she uses her hands to do anything. Anti-inflammatory medication seems to have no effect. At one point she develops some paresthesias in her right hand that go away after a week; at another she notices tremors in her thumb that come and go. By the time she seeks medical treatment for the injury it has spread to her other wrist for no apparent reason. It takes over two years before she spends whole days without pain. At three years since the initial injury, she still experiences symptoms from time to time in her daily life, especially after doing a massage. Her hands still feel different than they used to, as if they are not quite back to normal.

Tendinitis/Tenosynovitis

Tendinitis and tenosynovitis are inflammatory conditions of the tendon and tendon sheath respectively, as indicated by the suffix "-itis," meaning inflammation. These injuries are caused by tearing (strain) of tendon fibers or irritation to the tendon sheath. A tendon is made up of fibrous tissue that connects muscle to bone. A tendon sheath is a covering of connective tissue that envelops a tendon. Tendons that pass close to rigid structures, like those in the hand and foot, have sheaths to prevent bones and ligaments from wearing away at them, causing injury. The sheaths are filled with synovial fluid, which helps the tendons glide smoothly through them.

Tenosynovitis can be caused by a number of factors. Excessive repetitive motion of tendons may inflame the sheaths that surround them. Friction can also cause tenosynovitis when a sheath glides over a bone or joint. Scar tissue build-up in a tendon as a result of tendinitis may keep the tendon from gliding smoothly through its sheath, and the resulting rubbing of the scar tissue against the sheath can cause it to become inflamed. Thickening of the tendon or its sheath from inflammation or repetitive use (hypertrophy) creates even more rubbing/friction, and more inflammation. Awkward positioning may cause friction between the tendon, its sheath, and a bony structure that can produce inflammation in the sheath.

Whereas overuse is deemed a syndrome, a multi-faceted injury consisting of a number of different processes and reactions, tendinitis and tenosynovitis are thought to be more well-defined injuries in which inflammation is the main operating factor. It is the clear presence of inflammation that distinguishes these injuries from overuse syndrome. Among massage therapists, tendinitis/tenosynovitis are less frequent complaints than overuse syndrome. Some classic, common tendinitis and tenosynovitis injuries are: lateral epicondylitis (Tennis Elbow), an inflammation of the common tendinous origin of the forearm extensor muscles that results from a combination of overuse and misuse; medial epicondylitis (Golfer's Elbow), an inflammation of the common tendinous origin of the forearm flexors; and deQuervain's Thumb, an inflammation of the tendon sheath of the thumb abductors at the radiostyloid process.

Why do we spend so much time on tendons and tendon sheaths when discussing occupation-related upper limb injury? Muscle strain, or tearing of muscle fibers, can certainly happen as a result of giving massage, but it is a much less common occurrence than tendon strain. In fact, tendons are more commonly injured than most other structures of the body. Tendons attach muscle to bone near the fulcrum of movement (the joint), which is under great mechanical stress. If this stress is amplified by repetitive or improper use, the tendons are likely to tear.

Tendons are also poorly vascularized (few blood vessels) and poorly innervated (few nerve endings). With insufficient innervation, damage to the tendon is not felt as quickly as in muscle, so tears may happen before the nervous system can respond and ease tension on the tendon. With a small blood supply, tendons heal slowly, with potential for uneven scarring and the subsequent formation of adhesions. Since the scar tissue is weaker than the original tissue, the chances of reinjury are increased.

In contrast to overuse syndrome, which is characterized by slow, gradual onset, classic tendinitis and tenosynovitis are more often associated with traumatic onset, either in a single event, or with a sudden increase in activity over a short period of time. In a common scenario, someone goes out to play tennis after not playing for years, and at the end of five sets, the outside of the elbow is exquisitely painful and somewhat swollen. The more traumatic nature of the onset is consistent with the classic and marked inflammatory response that is seen in these injuries and is not seen in overuse syndrome. A traumatic onset may be precipitated in a part of the body that has been subject to repetitive stress. For example, a massage therapist will more likely develop lateral epicondylitis in his right arm after six hours spent playing tennis if he already has been overusing his forearm extensors in his massage work. An incipient or existing overuse injury in that area makes it more vulnerable to tendinitis.

Tenosynovitis may have a longer onset than classic tendinitis if overuse is the reason for the inflammation. Excessive repetitive motion can cause friction and/or hypertrophy of tendons, both of which can lead to inflammation in the tendon sheath. Tendinitis and tenosynovitis can become chronic if not allowed adequate healing time, or if the injury/reinjury cycle is set in motion.

The characteristic symptom of these injuries is localized pain ranging from mild to severe. Pain generally is worse with movement and better with rest. The more tendon fibers torn, the worse the pain and the longer the healing time. Pain may radiate distally or proximally. The affected area is often painful and hot to the touch. Swelling is also common. Redness is seldom visible, since the injury is deep enough to the skin to make redness imperceptible. Some loss of function may occur as a result of edema, pain, or build-up of scar tissue in a tendon. For example, if tendinitis occurs at a joint it may restrict movement, as in a trigger finger. Crepitus may be perceptible in the affected tendon as it moves through its sheath.

Although we have differentiated between overuse syndrome and tendinitis/tenosynovitis above, it is important to note that these distinctions are much clearer on paper than they are in actual practice. The percentage of cases that present with the classic symptoms and onsets described above is actually quite small: physicians put it at 5-10%. In the remaining 90% of patients, there is enough overlap in the presentation of the injury that it is no longer meaningful to call it by either name. If you can assess the relative contribution of overuse versus tendinitis, you will be better able to treat effectively.

Nerve Impingement Injury

Nerve plexuses and their roots can be compressed, irritated, pinched, or tugged on by the structures that surround them. Some assert that the basic cause of this impingement is overuse, and therefore categorize injuries like carpal tunnel syndrome and thoracic outlet syndrome as overuse or repetitive stress injuries. Nerves can be compressed by excessive use of muscles and tendons, causing hypertrophy or chronic hypertonicity. Inflammation of the nerve sheath from trauma to it or the joint it passes by, or inflammation resulting from overuse, can cause edema that can put pressure on nerves and impair their functioning. Scar tissue from a previous injury, traumatic or overuse, can compress or irritate a nerve. Impingement typically occurs in sites where nerves lie between hard structures (bone), or pass through or between softer, but still unyielding structures like muscle, tendon, ligament or fascia.

There are three nerves that innervate the forearm and hand: the median, the ulnar and the radial. These nerves can be entrapped at the wrist, elbow or shoulder. The median nerve may become impinged at the carpal tunnel of the wrist, or at the elbow by the pronator teres. At the elbow, the ulnar nerve may be entrapped in the cubital tunnel or in the condylar groove. The brachial plexus, the base of all three nerves and several others, may be compressed at the thoracic outlet. Radial nerve compression is less commonly a cause of occupation-related injury, although this nerve can become impinged near the elbow, creating symptoms similar to lateral epicondylitis (Tennis Elbow).

Nerve entrapment has a number of effects on the upper extremity:

1. Pressure on a nerve can cause inflammation and pain at the site of the entrapment. If left untreated, the mechanical pressure can cause damage to the nerve at that site.

2. Nerve compression can cause numbness and tingling distal to the site of the impingement.

3. Nerve compression can cause referred pain in the distal upper extremity. For this reason, it is often difficult to diagnose distal pain syndromes.

4. Nerve compression can reduce the amount of electrical impulses traveling through the nerve to the muscles. Tissues innervated distal to the compression site can become atrophied, weak, and prone to injury as a result.

5. Impingement at one site makes you more likely to develop a subsequent entrapment or injury at another site, usually distal to the original impingement site. This phenomenon, called double crush syndrome, is the result of the increase in neural (or nerve) tension created by the impingement. For example, an impingement somewhere along the median nerve, say at the elbow, would increase tension on the rest of the nerve, making you more vulnerable to carpal tunnel syndrome. Trauma or injury to the nerve can cause enough inflammation to create scar tissue in the nerve. The scar tissue can adhere the nerve to surrounding structures, causing compression of the nerve at that place.

Some physical therapists feel that upper extremity pain syndromes may be partially the result of neural tension, in addition to muscle strain or injury. Why does an increase in neural tension make you more susceptible to distal arm injury? Nerves have only a small amount of elasticity. The greater the tension on the nerve, the less elasticity it will have. When you bend your elbow, or wrist, or fingers while you are massaging, there will be less give in the nerve to allow for that motion. The bending motion will tug on the nerve, causing further irritation and inflammation, and injury.

Of all of the possible nerve impingement injuries, only carpal tunnel syndrome and thoracic outlet syndrome will be discussed in detail here. These are the two most common nerve impingement injuries among massage therapists. Muscle/tendon injury as a result of doing massage is more common among massage therapists than nerve impingement injury.

Carpal Tunnel Syndrome (CTS)

Because of the high visibility in the media of carpal tunnel syndrome as a result of computer keyboard overuse, CTS has become a catch-all term that is too often applied to any pain syndrome anywhere in the wrist area. There are many other injuries that can cause symptoms at the wrist. CTS, however, has quite a specific definition: it is impingement of the median nerve at the carpal tunnel, and nothing else!

The carpal tunnel is an oval passageway created by the rigid structures of the wrist (Illustration 1). The two rows of carpal bones in the wrist form an arch at the bottom of the tunnel. This arch forms the palm into a cup shape so we can hold objects. The top of the tunnel is formed by the transverse carpal ligament (flexor retinaculum). The bones and the ligament are rigid, so the space in the tunnel is fixed: it cannot expand to create more room. The size of the space varies from individual to individual.

Going through this fixed space are a number of soft tissue structures, namely the nine tendons of the forearm flexor muscles and the median nerve. CTS is a common injury because so many structures have to pass through such a small space. If anything happens to decrease the amount of space in the tunnel, pressure in the space increases and can cause the median nerve to be squeezed off. Even slight inflammation of a few of the flexor tendons from overuse (repetitive motion) can create enough edema to cause impingement of the median nerve. Overuse also can cause hypertrophy of the tendons or tendon sheaths, which can decrease the size of the tunnel and put further pressure on the median nerve.

CTS occurs when pressure on the median nerve cuts down on the volume of nerve impulses traveling through the nerve to and from the hand. It causes tingling at first, then loss of sensation and subsequent loss of function if severe and left untreated. Mechanical pressure on the nerve can damage the nerve tissue. Since nerve tissue is made up of permanent cells that cannot regenerate, advanced or untreated CTS can result in permanent nerve damage.

Positioning of the hand and wrist can also create pressure on the nerve. With the wrist in flexion for a sustained period of time, the median nerve can be compressed against the transverse ligament. Placing the wrist against an object like the edge of a desk for sustained periods can

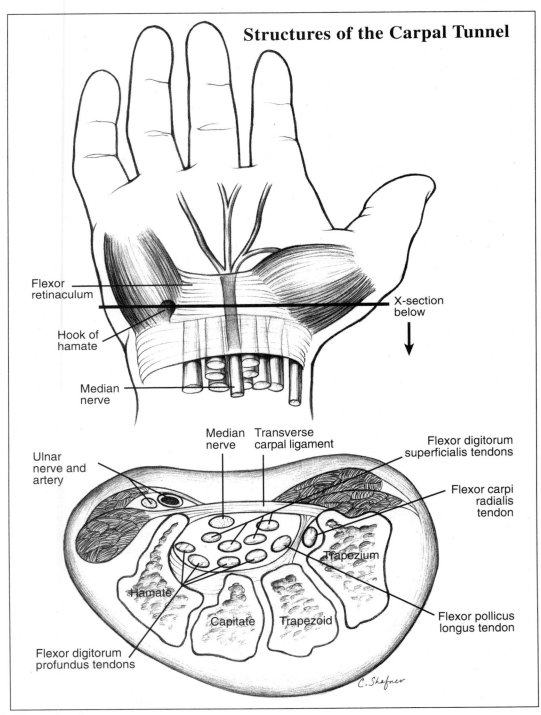

Structures of the Carpal Tunnel

Flexor retinaculum

Hook of hamate

Median nerve

X-section below

Ulnar nerve and artery

Median nerve

Transverse carpal ligament

Flexor digitorum superficialis tendons

Flexor carpi radialis tendon

Trapezium

Hamate

Capitate

Trapezoid

Flexor pollicus longus tendon

Flexor digitorum profundus tendons

C. Shefner

Illustration 1

also put mechanical stress on the median nerve, squashing it against the flexor retinaculum. The combination of wrist flexion and external pressure from an object can be especially detrimental.

Some members of the medical community speculate that women's ever-changing hormone levels may make them more susceptible than men to CTS, and to repetitive stress injuries in general. Another factor is the secretion of the hormone relaxin during menstruation, pregnancy, and breast feeding, which causes ligaments to become more lax. With decreased support from the ligaments, joints can become unstable, setting the stage for injury. Female massage therapists need to be particularly vigilant about self-care the week before they menstruate in order to avoid CTS. A small amount of relaxin is secreted during menstruation, which, along with fluid retention, can increase the risk of median nerve compression. During pregnancy, increased fluid volume and retention can increase pressure on the median nerve in the carpal tunnel, causing CTS. If you plan to do massage while you are pregnant, watch for the beginnings of CTS symptoms in the wrists and hands. Symptoms of CTS usually resolve after pregnancy, but any scar tissue that has built up from overuse and inflammation may still create problems. You can begin to see why CTS is more common in women than in men.

CTS is associated with several other conditions that involve fluid retention or fat deposition. Massage therapists with a history of thyroid disease or diabetes, or those taking oral contraceptives, have an increased risk of developing CTS.

The classic symptoms of CTS are pain, paresthesias and weakness of the hand. Pain is felt in the palmar aspect of the wrist radiating into the hand, particularly the palm, the thumb, index finger, third finger and the adjoining half of the ring finger (the innervation pattern of the median nerve). These fingers may loose some or all feeling and function. Paresthesias are experienced along the same innervation path. Shaking the hands can relieve these symptoms. It is common for CTS sufferers to be awakened by pain in the night, and to experience more pain in the morning than in the evening. CTS often affects both hands; if you currently have symptoms only in one hand, be on the lookout for the beginnings of symptoms in the other hand. A feeling of fullness or tightness in the wrists may precede other symptoms, and should be monitored carefully.

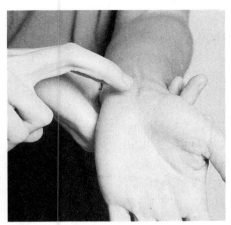

Photo 10

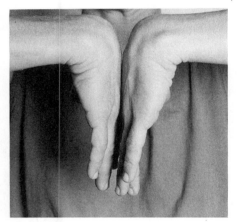

Photo 11

Like overuse syndrome, CTS tends to come on slowly and can be triggered by a sudden increase in workload or decrease in the time allowed between massages. Psychological stress is also a contributing factor.

Two tests are commonly used to check for CTS. They are easy to perform on clients and for yourself. To perform Tinel's Sign, tap firmly on the palmar side of the wrist where the hand begins, approximately in the center over the median nerve (Photo 10). If you elicit pain shooting into the hand, and/or numbness and tingling in the hand/fingers as you tap, this is a positive Tinel's Sign. For Phalen's Sign, put the backs of the hands together with the forearms straight out to the sides (Photo 11). Hold the position for one minute, or until you feel pain or discomfort. This position, with the wrists in 90 degrees of flexion, puts pressure on the carpal tunnel and the median nerve. If pain or paresthesias are felt in the wrist or hand, you have a positive Phalen's Sign. A positive Tinel's Sign or Phalen's Sign is highly suggestive of CTS; however, these tests are too crude to rely upon for a diagnosis when definitive treatment (i.e., surgery) is planned.

Take a moment here to consider your own wrists. Are they large, small, or in between? Persons with especially small wrists, and therefore small carpal tunnels, can be more prone to CTS. If you are a women, do you tend to retain water before or during your period? Are you planning to become pregnant? Any of these factors can make you more vulnerable to CTS.

Thoracic Outlet Syndrome (TOS)

The brachial plexus is a network of branches of spinal nerves C5-T1. In its course through the thorax, it passes between the anterior and middle heads of the scalene muscles and descends through the space between the first rib and the clavicle (Illustration 2). This area at the base of the neck is called the thoracic outlet. After the plexus passes through

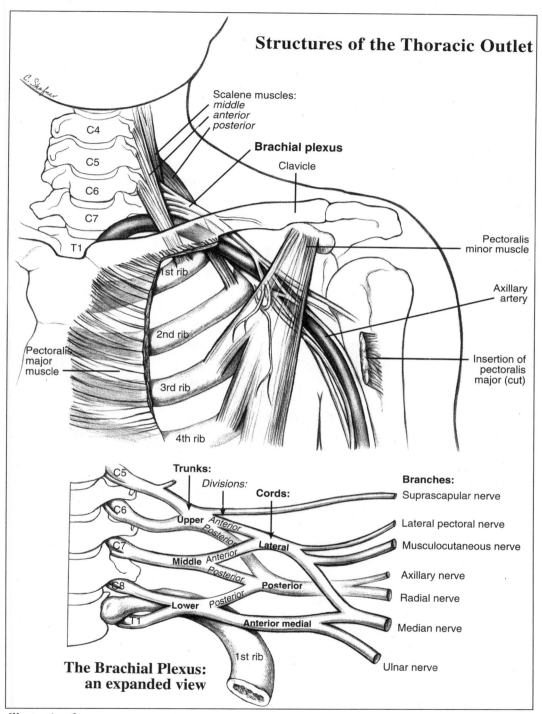

Structures of the Thoracic Outlet

Scalene muscles:
middle
anterior
posterior

Brachial plexus

Clavicle

C4
C5
C6
C7
T1

1st rib

2nd rib

3rd rib

4th rib

Pectoralis major muscle

Pectoralis minor muscle

Axillary artery

Insertion of pectoralis major (cut)

Trunks:

Divisions:

Cords:

Branches:

C5

C6

Suprascapular nerve

Lateral pectoral nerve

Upper *Anterior*
Posterior

Lateral

Musculocutaneous nerve

C7

Middle Anterior

Posterior

Posterior

Axillary nerve

Radial nerve

C8

Posterior

Lower

Anterior medial

Median nerve

T1

1st rib

Ulnar nerve

**The Brachial Plexus:
an expanded view**

Illustration 2

the thoracic outlet, it descends into the axillary region (armpit) and branches into the nerves of the arm, the most important of which are the radial, median and ulnar nerves.

The thoracic outlet is a small, confined area like the carpal tunnel, defined by bones on two sides and containing a number of other rigid structures. Abnormalities in any of these structures themselves, or in their position relative to each other, can cause the nerves of the plexus to be compressed and impinged. Thoracic outlet syndrome (TOS) refers specifically to impingement of nerves C8-T1 at the level of the thoracic outlet, which can create symptoms in the neck, shoulders, and hands. Compression of the axillary artery at the thoracic outlet may also be part of the syndrome.

The primary symptom of TOS is pain in the cervical region and suprascapular regions which may radiate down into the triceps, then the inner arm, the medial forearm and the ulnar side of the hand. The pain may be shooting or dull in nature, and may manifest simply as general arm pain. Diminished nerve impulses can cause paresthesias and, eventually, weakening and atrophy of distal muscles along the nerve route. Diminished blood flow to the arm caused by compression of the axillary artery can deprive the arm of the circulation needed to efficiently heal injuries. The ipsilateral hand may become cold or very pale as a result. Reduction in nerve impulses leads to a progressive decrease in dexterity and fine motor control. The posterior cervical muscles can go into spasm, causing the suboccipital muscles to contract as well. Some feel that contraction of these muscles can result in severe headaches.

In the early stages of TOS, the massage therapist may notice symptoms only while doing massage in the posture that caused the injury. In more advanced cases, symptoms may be present at any time, and may become constant. Pain is usually worse at night, and lessens during the daytime and with activity, except for those activities that trigger it.

Gradual onset is most common in TOS attributable to overuse. Repetitive motion in sustained poor postures has a cumulative effect over time, causing pressure on nerves C8-T1 of the brachial plexus.

In fact, poor posture is the primary cause of TOS. Sustained positions that change the angle of the clavicle to the first rib, or that bring the two bones closer to each other, can decrease the space in the thoracic outlet. House painters, carpenters, certain types of musicians, and hair stylists often get TOS from holding their arms raised for long periods as they work. Massage therapists tend to get TOS from working in a posture where the head is jutted forward and the shoulders are rounded. Women with shoulders that slant downward are more prone to TOS because the sloping of the shoulder decreases the angle between the first rib and the clavicle (once again, TOS seems to be more common in women than in men).

There are three common sites of C8-T1 nerve impingement that contribute to TOS:

1. Between the clavicle and the first rib, where tight scalenes can pull on the two bones and approximate them, or poor posture can tilt the first rib forward, compressing the nerves;
2. At the inter-scalene triangle, where muscular hypertonicity can squeeze the nerves, or spasm can raise the first rib and cause pinch nerves; and/or
3. In the pectoralis minor muscle, where hypertonicity and spasm can compress nerves against the second and third ribs;

Persons who are born with an extra rib above the first rib (a "cervical rib") are more prone to TOS. The presence of another bony structure in the already small and crowded thoracic outlet space can press on the nerves and cause injury. Very tight scalene muscles can cause, or be a contributing factor to TOS. If the scalenes are overcontracted, they can pull on the first rib. The resulting change in the position of the first rib can put pressure on the nerves. The nerves can be squeezed between the anterior and middle heads of the scalenes closer to the muscle belly if the muscle is hypertonic, hypertrophied or in spasm. Another muscle that can contribute to TOS is the pectoralis minor, which is often tight in people with rounded shoulders.

Roos' Sign is a useful test for TOS. Put your arms up with the elbows out to the side and the palms facing forward, like a traffic cop saying "Stop" with both hands (Photo 12). Keeping your arms in this position, open and close your hands quickly and continuously for three minutes. If during that time you start to feel numbness and/or tingling in the hands, or if your hands get very cold and/or white, it is possible that you have TOS to some degree. Remember that, like Tinel's Sign and Phalen's Sign for CTS, Roos' Sign is only *suggestive* of TOS. You will need to see a doctor for a complete and accurate diagnosis.

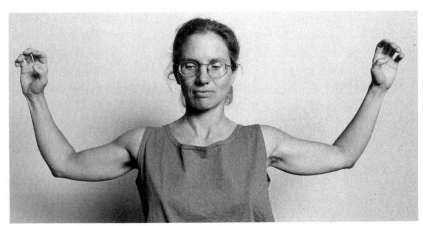

Photo 12

Now that we have discussed muscle/tendon and nerve impingement injuries, you may be convinced that you have one of these injuries. If you are already experiencing some of the symptoms mentioned in this chapter, stay calm and get yourself to a doctor who can diagnose your symptoms and get you on the road to recovery. There are many treatment options available to you if you are indeed injured. They are discussed in Chapter 8.

5

Preventing Injury by Changing Your Approach to Massage

Each massage therapist must develop a massage technique that allows him to use his body in an ergonomic, healthy fashion. Using good body mechanics helps you distribute stress evenly throughout the body instead of allowing it to accumulate in one area, which can lead to injury. Good body mechanics allow you to use the strength and momentum of the entire body to create motion that is flowing, even, relaxed and controlled. Any factor that interferes with the working of the body as a whole unit can put you at risk for injury.

This chapter discusses how to use your body in the most efficient possible manner as you massage. Your breathing, posture and positioning in relation to the client play an important role in your ability to prevent injury. Finding more natural, relaxed, and balanced ways to approach the physical work of massage will help you massage with less stress to your upper extremity and your body in general.

Most people would agree that the hands are the primary tool used in doing massage. However, to prevent injury effectively, and to heal when it occurs, you must examine much more than just the way you use your hands. The hands operate as part of a complex system that can easily be thrown off by many factors. Your posture, your breathing, and your emotional state can distort the natural, healthy use of the hands and increase your risk of injury. Monitoring these holistic aspects of your body as you do massage will help you avoid overstressing your hands and arms.

Breathing

Deep, regular breathing is an important, and often overlooked, component of good body mechanics. Breathing has a tremendous impact on your physical and emotional health. Conversely, the pattern of your breathing is affected by your physical position and your emotional state. Poor posture can make deep breathing difficult, especially if the chest is somewhat caved in. Often poor breathing is the result of unconscious tension: being uptight about doing a good massage, or paying attention more to the client's needs than your own, for example. When you are tense or under stress, you will tend to breathe shallowly, often from the chest instead of the diaphragm. You may even hold your breath at times without realizing it, especially when you are concentrating intensely. Many massage therapists breath shallowly or hold their breath as they work. Accumulated tension makes you more prone to injury not only physiologically, but also emotionally, since emotional tension interferes with your overall body awareness.

Body awareness must include breath awareness. You can learn to work with your breath as you massage by consciously reminding yourself to breath as you give a massage. Deep, conscious breathing almost instantly can counteract both emotional and physical tension. If you realize that your hands or arms are tense, take a deep breath from the diaphragm and blow it out. You will usually be able to see the muscular tension go out with the breath. Conscious breathing has the benefit of relaxing both you and your client. Your breathing reminds your client to breathe, and the work you do will have a deeper effect on him as a result. Chapter 7 contains some easy exercises that will help you get in the habit of deep, regular breathing.

Posture

The teaching of body mechanics for massage therapists has usually focused on being grounded and centered, and shifting your weight with your legs to help create movement and pressure with the arms. The knees are kept slightly bent, and the pelvis is kept in a neutral position. These are valid and useful concepts. The problem is that the emphasis is on the posture of the lower body, while most people have more trouble keeping their upper body in a healthy posture.

Unless the shoulder girdle is in neutral position, anything you do with your lower body will have little effect on your upper extremity. It is as though the upper body has been disconnected from the lower body. The musculature and joints of the upper extremity cannot respond to the motion of the rest of the body.

Most Americans have poor posture. We stand with our shoulders internally rotated, our chests caved in, and our heads jutted forward (Photo 13). In this posture, we lose all proximal support for the work we do with our arms. The work of the arms is meant to be supported by the larger, stronger muscles of the chest, shoulder, and back. The movement originates there, and that is the source of power for the arms.

The upper body and arm muscles are designed to work with the body in neutral position, with the joints aligned so there is an equal pull of muscles on

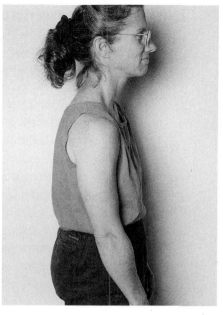

Photo 13

both the anterior and posterior side of the body. If you change this position by internally rotating the shoulders and caving in the chest, you end up over-stretching the muscles across the upper back and shortening the muscles in the chest and front of the shoulder. The result is a muscular imbalance that can contribute to injury. The upper back muscles become weak from disuse, and the chest and arm muscles become overcontracted and injured from overuse. It becomes impossible for the muscles to work efficiently to support the work of the shoulder girdle and the arm. The arm has to take up the slack, and ends up taking on much more work and stress than it was ever designed to withstand.

The arms are already overused from the activities of daily life. Typing, cooking, playing the piano, writing, doing the dishes -- all of these activities require us to hold our arms out in front of us, and then pronate the forearms so the palm of the hand is facing down. Massage is another activity done in this position, and can be a particularly strenuous one. The position in and of itself places considerable strain on the muscles of the arm, especially since many of us are already in a posture that prevents the larger muscles of the upper back and chest from helping out. To get these muscles back into a position where they can once again support the work of the arm, to reconnect them with the rest of the body, the shoulders need to be brought back into neutral. You can counteract the effects of bad posture by concentrating on moving as much from the back of the body as from the front.

The key to re-engaging these muscles is scapular stabilization. The scapula is the structural and functional link between the spine and the arm. The muscles of the chest, back, and upper arm attach to it. Stabilizing the scapula involves getting the scapula back into neutral so that the stress coming through the arm can be distributed evenly between the chest and the upper back. When this is achieved, the muscles of the arms no longer have to work as hard, because they are no longer doing all the work. Scapular stabilization also allows you to connect the work of the arms to the rest of the body, so you can use your whole body to create motion and pressure.

Stabilizing the scapula requires two steps: returning the shoulders to neutral and lifting up the chest to restore the normal amount of kyphotic curve to the thoracic spine, and bringing the rib cage, cervical spine and head into alignment with the rest of the body. Stand sideways in front of a full length mirror with your feet a comfortable distance apart (no more than shoulder width). Think of your legs as the roots of a tree, firm and strong. Keeping the knees slightly bent, shift your weight gently from side to side to find your center of gravity. You will want to maintain your center of gravity at all times while you work, so that you are never off-balance. Working upward from this firm base, the next step is your trunk. Like the trunk of a tree, the trunk of your body is the largest, most stable part of your anatomy. To keep the lower part of the trunk in alignment, make sure your pelvis and low back are in a neutral position: neither sticking out in the back nor tucked under. To help you get the feel of this position, think about "lengthening" your lumbar spine, letting it relax into its natural curvature as opposed to an exaggerated "sway back" posture.

At the top of the trunk, the upper back and the shoulders need to be aligned with the rest of the body. Relax your shoulders and lift your chest upward until your shoulders, rib cage, and head line up with the rest of your body. Lift just enough to get back into a comfortable, relaxed, neutral position -- do not stick your chest out, nor push your shoulders back unnaturally. Use your breath to counteract any tension in your shoulders. Check your alignment in the mirror. Let your arms hang naturally by your sides (Photo 14).

With the joints and muscles of your body in good alignment, you can use the upper back to help move the arms, instead of using the muscles of the arm by themselves. Try this exercise to see how it feels to lift your arms into abduction using the muscles of the upper back and chest equally to produce the motion. Keep your arms straight, and concentrate on feeling your rhomboids and lower trapezii contract to lift the arms to the sides, with some assistance from the deltoid and supraspinatus muscles on top of the shoulder (Photo 15). You may need to help a little at first by pinching your shoulder blades together slightly as you begin lifting your arms. You should have a feeling of openness in your chest and stability in your shoulders and upper back as you lift. Make sure you keep breathing to counteract tension. Return your arms to your sides. Repeat this exercise with flexion. Lift your arms straight in front of you, once again pinching your shoulder blades together, using your rhomboids and lower trapezii to initiate the movement.

Incorporating scapular stabilization into your massage technique takes some practise. To get the feeling of using the entire body in each stroke, you can start with a simple exercise that illustrates the difference between working with scapular stabilization (with your scapulas engaged and neutral) and working without it. It also uses the principle of joint alignment discussed in Chapter 2: the body is under the least stress when the bones and joints are lined up with one another.

Stand at the side of your massage table with your feet a comfortable distance apart. Bend your legs and move slightly from side to side to find your center of gravity. If you prefer to work with one

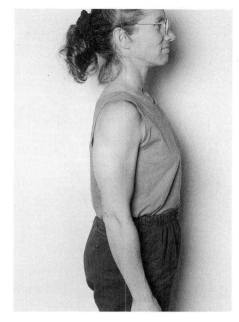

Photo 14

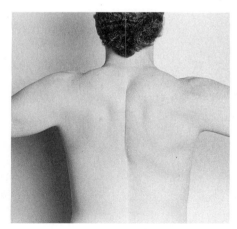

Photo 15

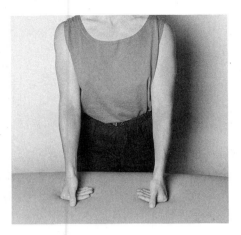

Photo 16

foot behind the other when you are at the side of the table, do so, but make sure your weight is distributed evenly over both of your feet. "Lengthen" your spine (let your pelvis and low back assume a neutral position), then stabilize your scapulas by lifting your chest upward. Make a loose fist with both hands. Keeping your arms straight, lean forward and rest the front of your fist on the table (Photo 16). The broad, flat surface of your fist creates greater stability, which will help ensure that stress is distributed evenly. Check your scapulas to make sure they are still in neutral position. Keep breathing!

Keeping your joints lined up on top of each other, bend your knees slightly and let your fists sink into the padding of the table. Be sure to keep your hands soft, but still in a fist. Don't *push* the fists into the table with the arms. Don't let your arms move independently from the rest of the body in any way. Breathe! Think of the arms as dead sticks: able to stay firm to absorb movement generated by the upper body, but not able to move unless the upper body makes them move. If you know CPR, you will recognize this concept from the way chest compressions are performed. Let your body move as one unit, so that your body weight can go into your arms through your upper back and shoulders to create the downward motion that increases the pressure. Straighten your knees a bit and see how the pressure gradually and evenly lessens. Using this technique, you can achieve any degree of pressure, from very light to very deep. Experiment with applying different degrees of pressure using this technique.

Now try the same exercise without scapular stabilization. Allow your shoulders to internally rotate, and the chest to cave in slightly. You will notice that you are more inclined now to use the arms to create motion and pressure, and that it is difficult for the upper extremity to work in concert with the rest of the body. Without proximal support, the arm can easily become unstable and wobbly. When this happens, the arm muscles must work harder to control the arm and keep it stable. The goal is to let the muscles of the arm rest as much as possible by letting the alignment of the joints and the control of the rest of the body create the strokes and the pressure. This concept can be used in many of the moves you do in your massages.

Using scapular stabilization in your massage work has added benefits. Scapular stabilization will make your strokes and pressure more even and controlled. The large, strong muscles can regulate heavier pressure and larger movements much more easily and smoothly than the smaller muscles of the arms alone. The healthier posture also promotes good breathing by opening the chest. Pressure is taken off blood vessels and nerves, allowing proper blood/lymph flow and innervation to the arms. Injuries like carpal tunnel syndrome and thoracic outlet syndrome can be prevented and rehabilitated by using scapular stabilization.

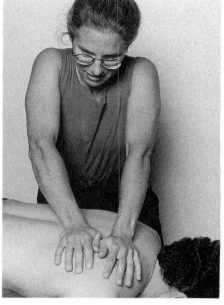

Photo 17

As you work, try to develop awareness of the position of your scapulas. After a while, this will become automatic. In the meantime, stop every once in a while and ask yourself "where are my shoulders?" You may find that they have raised up into the "wearing your shoulders like earrings" position (Photo 17). This may be the result of tension, or lack of upper body strength, or simply careless posture. Repetitively raising the shoulders as you work can cause rotator cuff injury in itself! Take a deep breath and let your shoulders fall back down gently. If they have rolled back into internal rotation, lift your chest and lengthen your spine before you resume your work. A neutral shoulder position may feel odd or difficult to maintain at first, since most persons have very weak, stretched-out rhomboids and lower trapezii. With practice and strengthening (see exercises in Chapter 7), you will soon find the position more natural. To maintain good health and prevent injury, you should try to make this posture part of your everyday life.

Positioning

The healthiest working position is one that allows you to remain upright. Your arms should be a comfortable distance in front of your body, and the client should be close enough to you that you do not have to lean to reach him. In upright position, you can use your body to proximally support the work of your arms. Your work is right in front of you, within easy reach. If at any time you notice that you have moved out of this position, there are two ways to get back into it: either move the client (or ask him to move), or move yourself.

If you are standing at the side of the table, work only on the side of the client that is near you. Do not reach across the client to work on the other side; rather, walk over to that side and work there. Your client will tend to position herself in the exact center of the table, especially if she is on her stomach with her face in the face cradle. There is nothing wrong with asking your client to move over more to the side so she is closer to you. Make sure that your table is built securely enough that it will not move or begin to tip. You may want to organize your massage to address one side of the body at a time, so you and the client can stay on one side for a while and then switch to the other. If she is supine and you want to work on her upper body, you can have her lie diagonally across the table so her upper body is closer to you.

Some strokes, like long effleurage or friction strokes, can cover an area of several feet within one stroke. For example, when executing a deep friction stroke of the entire erector spinae group you might start at the base of the neck and cover the entire length of the back down to the iliac crest in one long stroke. If you stand at your client's head to do the stroke, you will have to start leaning over the client by the time you get halfway down his back (even if you have very long arms). The more you lean, the more your arms will have to work without proximal support. Try instead to work from the side, stay upright, and walk along with your stroke. Take small steps and move along the side of the table, so that your body propels the stroke forward. "Walking the arm" in this way is effective for addressing the length of the back, or the anterior leg and thigh, particularly if your client has a long torso or long legs.

Standing at the client's side and working along the length of the body creates a tendency to twist your body into an unnatural position and encourages you to ulnar or radially deviate your wrists (Photo 18). Try to stand at the side of the table and work perpendicularly to the client as much as possible when you massage. In this position, you will be able to keep your wrists straight and your body upright. "Wringing" is an excellent technique that is done in this position.

The client can lie on the massage table in one of three positions while you work on her: prone, supine, and side-lying. You can also work with your client seated in an on-site chair. You will find that strokes and techniques are often more effective and easier to perform in one position than in another. Take advantage of the opportunities each position affords you. Experiment with your clients in all four positions, and find out which of your techniques work best in each position. Learn to work *with* the position, not against it. As a general rule, work on the posterior side of the body when the client is prone, and the anterior side of the body when the client is supine. Do not do techniques in one position that could be more comfortably done in a different position. For example, working on the back while the client is supine requires you to get your hands underneath your client and press upward, a very stressful move for you. Instead, get the client into a side-lying, prone, or seated position, where the back is stretched out in front of you and you have more choices of less-stressful ways to approach it.

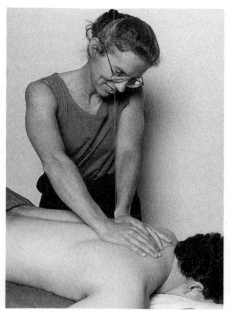

Photo 18

Work on the client in whatever position is best for *you*, unless that position causes the client pain or discomfort. If your choice of positioning is limited by the client's comfort, you will have to do only those techniques that you can do comfortably in the positions the client can tolerate. Forcing yourself to do techniques that are awkward in a given position can put you at risk for injury. Chapter 6 includes recommendations for specific techniques that can be done easily in each lying position.

Incorporating Motion and Variety Into Your Massage

The massage therapists who are able to practice for many years with little to no injury have a few noticeable characteristics in common. Two principles govern the way they work: motion and variety. They keep moving as they work, never spending more than a minute or so in one position or posture. They walk around their client as they work. Massaging a back, they stand at the client's head one moment, then walk over to stand at her shoulder, then her side. They are constantly adjusting their position in relation to the client to achieve the optimum posture and leverage to do their techniques. They change technique and hand/arm position frequently. First they may use a fist, then change to an open hand, then to a few fingers together. Each hand position lasts no more than a few strokes, then it's on to a new one to avoid too much repetitive motion. Frequently changing the part of the hand or arm you use keeps any one set of muscles from being overused and overstressed.

To reinforce your self-awareness, have a colleague watch you as you massage. Do you stand for long periods in one place, or do you move around your client? Do you do many of the same kind of stroke before changing to a different stroke? Are most of your strokes done with one part of your hand? For example, do you use your thumbs during 50% of the massage, or do you use your flat palm to the exclusion of any other part of your hand? You might also ask a third colleague to videotape you as you massage, or videotape yourself using a tripod. Then watch the tape and evaluate your massage. As you develop awareness of the way you work, you can start incorporating more movement and variety into your massages. Needless to say, it takes practice to develop the confidence and flexibility to work in this manner. It is definitely a model to emulate in your effort to stay injury-free.

Re-Organizing Your Massage Technique

Most therapists' massage technique consists of 70-80% small, fine movements and 20-30% large, broad motions. Many therapists feel obligated to work almost exclusively on small areas where they find adhesions, trigger points, pain, or injury. Many clients have enough of these problem spots to fill ten massages. The therapist often tries to treat as many of these spots as possible in one session. This approach has two potentially harmful effects. First, the client is overtreated. Too much spot work can cause nausea, dizziness, and grogginess, as well as the feeling that one has been poked and prodded mercilessly. The client should feel good after a massage, not pummeled! This excessive fine work also is hard on the massage therapist. It is difficult to use the large muscles of the back or the momentum of the body when one is working on small areas. Instead, therapists end up using the hand, fingers, or thumbs without proximal support. If spot work comprises the majority of your massages, you can easily overuse the small muscles of the arms and hands.

Massage training programs teach many techniques for treating every part of the body. For the anterior thigh, for example, you probably were taught a number of different techniques for each of the four quad muscles. Once you are out of school, you may think that you have to use as many of these techniques as possible in each massage. This kind of thinking can lead you to treat every inch of the anterior thigh of every client, even if the client is not having any trouble at all with that area. A few nice, broad, medium-depth effleurage strokes on the anterior thigh will incorporate this part of the body into the massage while saving your hands at the same time. The client will not miss the small work on the thigh, since he probably has other areas that have a more pressing need for your attention.

Large, broad, gentle strokes serve another important purpose as well: they aid in lymphatic drainage of the area. Part of the goal of massage is to help move accumulated toxins and waste products out of the muscles. Broad, light strokes used every few minutes between treatment techniques gently sweep the lymph fluid away from the affected area, moving toxins and waste back toward the general circulation where they can be processed and excreted. Breaking up your spot work with more general lymphatic drainage strokes is good for your client and easier on your hands.

Treating specific areas of tension or pain can be accomplished in many ways other than by applying pressure or friction to a specific area. Digging at a spot can cause muscle guarding, making the area even more tense, the opposite of the desired outcome. Some clients actually respond badly to intense spot work. If someone is already in pain, being caused more pain is not helpful. Massaging the general area using light to moderate pressure can be very effective in treating pain and injury. Increasing circulation, lymph flow, and muscular relaxation have a tremendously therapeutic effect on healing. You will do your clients a service by educating them about the benefits of less intrusive, less specific treatment work.

If your massages are too heavily weighted on small techniques, think about incorporating more large, broad strokes in your work. Remember that massage is a holistic method of healing; the most effective massages address the entire body, not just a few spots. Addressing the whole body reminds your client that he is more than just an injured shoulder or a sore back. This change in attitude can significantly affect how well he progresses in his treatment. Strike a balance between small techniques and broader strokes in your work. To maintain a long, healthy career, your massages should be comprised of not more than 40% small techniques; even fewer than that would be best.

Optimizing your body mechanics and your overall approach to massage will set you on the road to career longevity and upper extremity health. However, you must also examine the specific massage techniques you use for potentially harmful habits. In Chapter 6, you will learn how to modify some techniques and find alternates for others so you can reduce stress to your upper limbs.

6

Preventing Injury by Changing Specific Massage Techniques

Whether you are already injured or perfectly healthy, you should take a look at the techniques you use when doing massage to make sure you are not overstressing your hands and arms. Remember the primary rule: *if it hurts, don't do it.* If you are experiencing symptoms of injury, most likely something you are doing as you perform massage is causing those symptoms. Until you stop doing whatever that is, you will continue to injure yourself, and your symptoms will not go away. You should also stop doing anything that just feels uncomfortable or awkward, since these feelings are a good indication that what you are doing might eventually cause pain and injury. Changing the way you do massage *before* your body sends you the pain signal can short-circuit the injury process.

Many massage therapists become injured by performing techniques that are excessively stressful to their upper extremities. You can avoid overuse by becoming aware of how much you use any one part of your arm in your massages. Then you can reduce that usage by finding alternative strokes that use different parts of the arm. This chapter describes alternative techniques that can help you prevent overuse.

Harmful techniques either overuse one part of the upper limb, or use a particular part in an unstable position. Instability is troublesome because it can lead to unnatural positioning, one of the

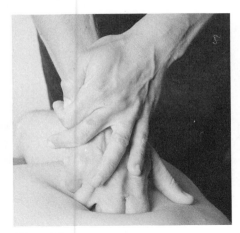

Photo 19

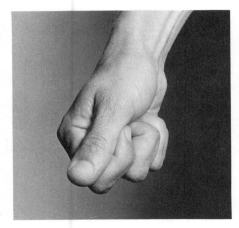

Photo 20

main factors that contributes to massage-caused injury. Avoid using any technique that puts the arms and/or hands in positions that are hard to control or cause the arm or hand to wobble. Use parts of the hand or arm that are broad and flat, like the forearm, the front of the fist, or the knuckles. These are the most stable. The thumb and the fingers are the most unstable to use, since they tend to buckle and wobble when pressure is applied.

You can enhance stability by reinforcing your hands, wrists, and fingers. The more stable the wrist or finger joints, the less the muscles have to work to keep the joints in alignment, thus taking stress off them. The added stability distributes stress more evenly. It also allows the muscles to relax more, since they no longer have to work so hard to maintain stable positioning.

There are many simple techniques for reinforcing your hands and fingers. Use your free hand to enhance stability at the wrist (Photo 19). Use two fingers at a time, never just one, to create more stability. To keep the thumb from buckling and wobbling when you apply pressure, make a relaxed fist, and let the index finger wrap slightly around the thumb (Photo 20). When using a flat palm, place the other palm on top of it. Keep the bottom hand soft and relaxed, so it can palpate properly. Good palpation requires only a small amount of pressure: the heavier the pressure, the more you lose sensitivity in your fingers. Think of the bottom hand as the palpating hand, and the upper one as the power hand, the one that propels and creates the pressure of the stroke. This same technique can be used with the fingertips.

Techniques Specific to Parts of the Upper Extremity

The rest of this chapter describes specific techniques in more detail.

Thumbs

If you use the thumb as a pressure device, a purpose it was not meant to serve, you are likely to injure it. A massage therapist's thumbs are often the first part of her body to become injured from overuse. It makes sense to avoid using the thumbs whenever possible. There are many other ways to use the hands and arms that can take the place of thumb work. One common use of the thumb is to create direct pressure on a small spot, for example a trigger point. Massage therapists like to use the thumb for this kind of treatment because they can use it both to palpate and to treat. There is nothing wrong with using the thumb to palpate. Palpation should be done lightly, otherwise your thumb or fingers will become less sensitive. Once you have found the spot you would like to treat, mark it with your thumb, place your elbow at that spot, and apply pressure with the elbow (see below for proper use of the elbow). You can follow the same steps using two knuckles together to apply the pressure while reinforcing the wrist with the other hand (Photo 19).

You may feel that a few of the techniques you do with your thumb are so effective that you are not willing to give them up, especially if you cannot find adequate alternatives for them. There may be some areas of the body that you may feel are best approached with the thumb and would be endangered or unreachable with any other technique. You can continue to use your thumbs in these cases if you stop overusing your thumbs at other times in your massages. Set a limit for how much you will use your thumbs in any one massage. For example, limiting yourself to using your thumbs for five minutes or less in each massage may make it possible to keep your thumbs healthy.

The healthiest way to use the thumb is to keep it supported and in line with the rest of the arm. The technique shown in Photo 21 is acceptable, as long as the base of the thumb (the thenar eminence) stays in contact with the client's body and pressure is not applied exclusively with the tip of the thumb. Photo 20 (above) shows a position in which

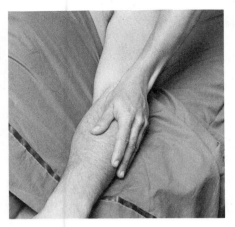

Photo 21

you can apply direct pressure with the thumb that at least supports the thumb with the index finger and fist, and lines it up with the rest of the arm.

Nonetheless, it is preferable not to use the thumb for direct pressure. If you are already experiencing pain or other symptoms of injury or impending injury in your thumbs, you will need to stop using them completely until they have healed. Explore other options for creating direct pressure, including using the elbow (see below), even if you are uninjured. The process of discovery can be very creative and fun!

Fingers

The fingers are also quite flexible, which makes them unstable and easy to injure. Individually, the fingers are weak. There are two joints in each finger, and the small muscles of the finger have to work very hard to stabilize these joints. The finger also needs to be stable at the junction of the hand to be able to work with the rest of the hand, and the wrist must be stable to allow the power of the arm and shoulder to reach the fingertips. While you are applying pressure, you must use a great deal of muscular tension to keep all of these joints stable at the same time. The extensor muscles of the forearm tend to become hypertonic and overtaxed when the fingertips are used repetitively to apply pressure in massage. Reinforcing the wrist with the other hand is helpful, but still does not provide enough stability in the finger joints.

The safest thing to do is to avoid using the fingertips in doing massage. Certainly if you are having pain in your fingers or in the extensor muscles of the forearm you will have to stop using this technique. As with the thumbs, if you are not injured and you feel you must do a few techniques with the fingertips, limit yourself to a few minutes in each massage.

There are many alternatives to working with the fingertips. As with the thumb, massage therapists like to use their fingertips because they are very sensitive for palpation. You can still use the fingertips for palpation; just don't use them to apply pressure. The ulnar side of the hand can create pressure (Photo 22). The front of the fist can provide good, even, strong pressure, especially if the wrist is reinforced with the other hand. A flat palm can be an alternative, although it does put some strain on the forearm flexors. You will need to be careful about the position of your wrist if you apply pressure with a flat palm.

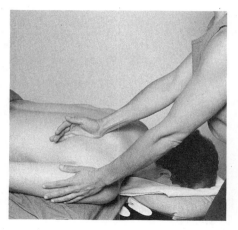

More and more massage therapists are now using hand-held massage tools to create pressure instead of using their thumbs or fingertips. If these are used carefully and sensitively, the client often will not even realize that you are using a tool instead of your hand. These tools are available from the same sources that sell massage supplies. They come in a number of shapes and sizes, with names

Photo 22

like "The Knobble®," "Index Knobber," and "T-Bars." Some therapists like to use stones made out of marble or semiprecious gems because of the healing properties attributed to them.

Using tools does not avoid all problems, unfortunately. They must be gripped with the palm and/or fingers, and the repetitive gripping can also cause overuse injury. For some therapists, gripping causes fewer adverse effects than using their thumbs or fingertips. Others will find gripping more problematic. Experiment with different tools to find out whether they work for you.

Hands

Keep your hands soft and relaxed as you work. Tense hands can be the result of incorrect posture, holding your breath as you work, or feelings of stress, uncertainty, or lack of confidence. Constant isometric contraction can cause an overuse syndrome of the intrinsic muscles of the hand in some cases, and sets the stage for injury in all cases. Tense, stiff, and unyielding hands also feel bad to your client. You want to relax your client, not transmit your tension to her. Let your hands mold to the individual contours of your client's body.

Forearms

The best way to save your hands is to avoid using them altogether whenever possible. The forearms can be extremely effective tools in

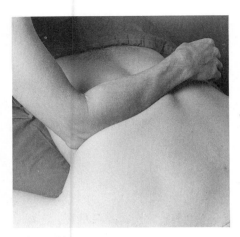

Photo 23

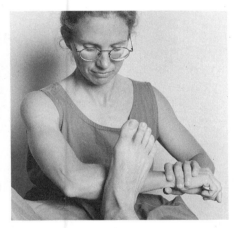

Photo 24

doing massage work, and can replace the hands in many techniques. A Hawaiian massage form called Lomi Lomi uses the forearms and elbows almost exclusively to do massage. Some of the Lomi Lomi techniques can be easily adapted for use in your massages. Use them as alternative strokes to replace techniques that use the hands.

The basic Lomi Lomi stroke, "ironing," uses the forearm to compress and lengthen a broad area of tissue (Photo 23). Another effective stroke called "circling" lengthens and lifts the tissue by pushing upward in small circles. Circling can replace other petrissage strokes that use the hands. Lomi Lomi strokes are very effective for addressing broad areas like the back, the gluteals, the anterior or posterior thigh, the posterior calf, and the bottom of the foot (Photo 24). You can apply pressure either with the ulna (the side of the forearm) or the flexor muscles (the volar side of the forearm). The ulna provides more specific pressure, while the volar forearm provides more general, broad pressure. In forearm work, there is a tendency to clench the fist in response to tension, especially when you are new to the technique. If your hand becomes tense, relax it both consciously and with your breathing.

You may find that forearm techniques are too rough for thin clients who have prominent bones. Experiment with using the forearm on different parts of the body in different ways to see what works best for you and your client. Be sure to use plenty of lubrication for forearm techniques, and maintain communication with your client about pressure and comfort.

Elbows

· Your elbows can be wonderful massage tools if they are used carefully. It takes practice to become comfortable with using the elbow to provide pressure. It is important when using the elbows to support them by stabilizing your scapula (see Chapter 5) in order to regulate pressure and keep the elbow in the right location. Without proximal support, the arm can be hard to control, and you can hurt your client by applying too much pressure or by sliding onto nerves, blood vessels, or bones.

To apply direct pressure with the elbow, use your fingers or thumb to palpate for adhesions and trigger or pressure points. When you find a spot you want to treat, stabilize your scapula and place the elbow on top of the spot. Keeping the upper arm vertical, create pressure by sinking in with your entire body, bending your knees if necessary, until the desired depth is reached. Relax your hands as you work with your elbow. Work with only one elbow at a time, using the other hand to make sure you are away from any delicate soft tissue structures or bones. For example, when treating a spot next to the spinal column, keep the free hand on the spinous processes to make sure you avoid them.

You can also use your elbow with the forearm horizontal (Photo 25). This technique can be an effective alternative to using the hands to create a long stroke down the erector spinae muscles of the back.

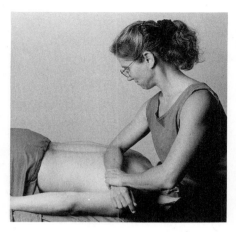

Photo 25

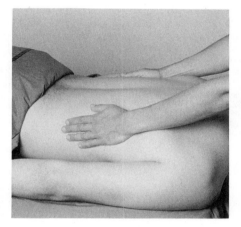

Photo 26

Wrists

To protect the wrists from injury, you must keep them as straight as possible as you work. Repetitive radial and ulnar deviation of the wrist, with or without pressure, can cause injury. Ulnar deviation has become part of one of the most basic Swedish massage strokes, namely effleurage to spread oil on the client's back. The therapist stands at the head and spreads oil on the back with his flat palms. As his hands reach the low back, he ulnar deviates them to spread oil to the sides as he comes

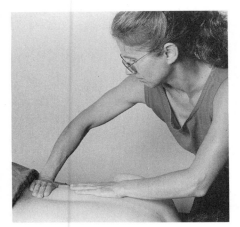

Photo 27

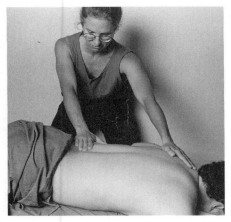

Photo 28

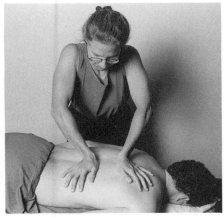

Photo 29

back up. There is no need to ulnar deviate to encompass the sides of the back. Simply keep the wrist straight as you come down to the side from the low back, and make sure they stay straight as you move up the sides toward the head (Photo 26). Remember also that you do not have to spread oil from the neck going down. You can spread it from the side, which allows you to keep your wrists perfectly straight.

Here is a simple way to straighten out your hands if you notice they are in ulnar or radial deviation (Photo 27). Keep your hand where it is on the client, and "walk" the arm straight by moving around the client until the hand and arm are once again aligned (Photo 28). This trick will help you avoid returning to the previous unhealthy posture by giving you a different place to stand so that your wrists can remain straight as you do the technique.

Ulnar deviation can happen as a result of keeping the arms constantly pronated when doing massage (see Chapter 7). This constant pronation causes excessive stress of the forearm muscles. The shoulders and arms try to compensate for this stress by internally rotating at the shoulder and abducting the arms with the elbows going out to the sides. This positioning causes the hands to go into ulnar deviation as you work (Photo 29). Computer operators often end up in this position; it sets them up to be injured. Be aware of this chain of events and try to counteract it if you see it happening. Bring the elbows back in toward the body, allowing the wrists to straighten out.

Hyperflexion and hyperextension of the wrists should also be avoided, especially with pressure. In these positions, structures of the wrist are compressed and can be damaged. Hyperflexion and hyperextension can happen when you use the flat part of the fist (Photo 30) or a flat palm (Photo 31).

A table that is too high or too low can put your wrist in one of these positions. If you notice this happening, adjust the table height until the wrist is straight once again. A hydraulic or electric table is invaluable for making this kind of quick adjustment (see Chapter 2). Going back to spreading oil: when you come around to the sides of the neck, you can easily hyperextend the wrist (Photo 32). If you must do this part of the stroke, use very little pressure when you get to the neck and keep your hands moving so your wrists are hyperextended for only a moment. You can always apply oil to the neck standing at your client's side where it is easier to keep your wrists straight.

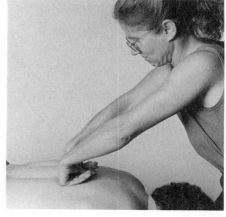

Photo 30

Working With the Client's Position

As discussed in Chapter 5, positioning your client to your best advantage can help you reduce stress in your massage work. Each position -- prone, supine, side-lying, and seated -- places the therapist at a different angle to the client's body. Each provides unique opportunities to access parts of the client's body while allowing the therapist to work comfortably.

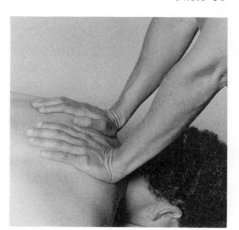

Photo 31

Sidelying Position

Of the three possible lying positions, sidelying position is the most often overlooked and underutilized by massage therapists. Those therapists who seldom use the sidelying position do themselves a disservice, since it is arguably the best position in which to work. In this position, one entire side of the client's body is turned toward the therapist and can be positioned close to the edge of the table to be within easy reach of the therapist. Working in this position, the therapist can remain upright, in good

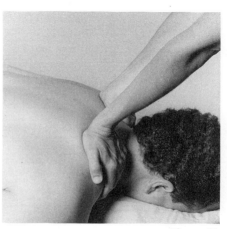

Photo 32

81

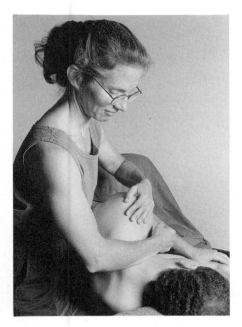

Photo 33

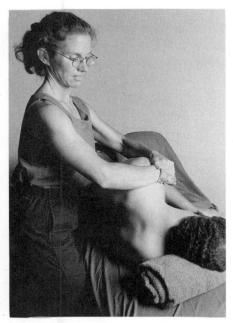

Photo 34

body alignment, with her wrists straight, cutting down on stress to her arms and hands. Forearm techniques work very well in sidelying position. With proper bolstering, most clients find sidelying position more comfortable than prone or supine position, especially during pregnancy or with back pain.

Muscles located on the side of the body that would be difficult to massage in prone or supine position are very accessible and easy to work on in sidelying position. You can use your forearms extensively to work with these muscles in this position to give your hands a rest and to achieve a broad, even stroke. This position gives you the opportunity to tie together the different sections of the body, flowing consecutively from the neck down into the back into the gluteals and down to the thigh.

A number of specific techniques work quite well on the lateral muscles with the therapist standing behind the client:

Side of the neck: Place the forearm at the occiput, and stroke slowly down the trapezius to the end of the shoulder (Photo 33). Be careful to avoid the delicate structures of the anterior and posterior neck triangle as you come down the neck. Check in regularly with your client to determine appropriate pressure. Hold your wrist with your free hand and lean back, using your body weight, not your arms, to give the client a good upper trapezius stretch (Photo 34).

Latissimus dorsi, teres major, serratus anterior: With your client's arm over his head, place your forearm just below the rib cage near the latissimus origin. Apply moderate pressure and move evenly up toward the shoulder joint, encompassing the teres major and serratus muscles as you go (Photo 35). If your client's ribs are not too prominent, use the Lomi Lomi circling technique at the broadest part of the muscles. Continue up to the head of the humerus.

Medial border of scapula: When your client lies on her side, her superior scapula will likely wing out, making the medial border accessible for massage. Use your elbow or two or more knuckles together to push upward and under the scapula. You may find this technique easier to do if you get on your knees on the floor (Photo 36).

Erector spinae muscles of the superior side: These muscles will bulge out slightly in this position due to gravity. With the muscles more prominent, you can get at them more easily. Try using your forearm and elbow to create an even friction stroke from the base of the neck to the iliac crest, keeping the hand relaxed and the arm perpendicular (90 degree angle) to the client's spine (Photo 37).

Quadratus lumborum: Sidelying is the only position that gives you access to the quadratus lumborum. If there is enough room between the client's last rib and the edge of the hip, you can use your elbow to sink down and apply direct pressure to the quadratus lumborum (Photo 38). You can create more room between the last rib and the hip by placing a pillow or folded towel under their opposite side just above the hip.

Gluteal muscles: Use the forearm in ironing or circling motions on the gluteals. Ask the client to lean forward a bit to expose more of the posterior gluteals: use the elbow around the lateral border of the sacrum (carefully avoiding bone) and to apply direct pressure to adhesions and trigger points. From the gluteals you can sweep directly into the:

Iliotibial band: Sidelying is the ideal position to use for treating the IT band. Use the forearm in ironing or circling motions as you move from the hip down the IT band to the knee.

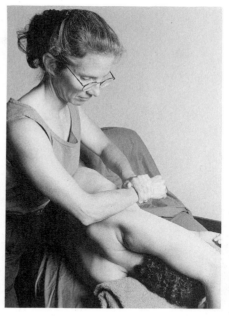

Photo 35

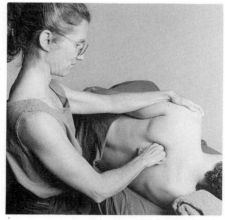

Photo 36

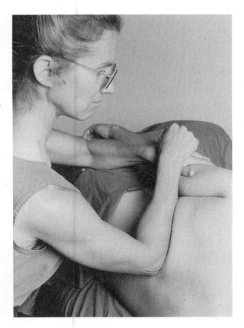

Photo 37

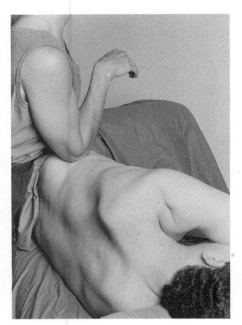

Photo 38

Tensor fasciae latae: This muscle can be easily accessed in sidelying position. Ask the client to lean backward toward you a bit so you don't have to lean over to reach the TFL. Use the forearm for broad friction, and the elbow for spot work.

Supine Position

To maintain healthy alignment of your body with the client in supine position, work only on the anterior aspect of the body. The one exception is the IT band, which can be worked with your fist. Brace your elbow against your hip and move your body to create the pressure (Photo 39). Be sure not to tense your fist as you do this move. You can use your forearm on the IT band if you reposition the client so that his knee and hip are flexed and his foot is resting on the table.

Supine is a good position for working on the arms. Stand on the side of the table, facing your client's head, to address the length of the arm. Avoid foot work in supine position; you may however, use your forearm to apply pressure to the foot to increase ROM in flexion and extension.

Prone Position

Concentrate on the posterior aspect of the body in prone position, again with the exception that the IT band remains accessible in this position. In prone position, the bottom of the feet can be massaged using your forearm and elbow, giving you an opportunity to rest your hands. The backs of the legs can be massaged with your forearms. To avoid leaning over the client to massage the calfs, bend her leg into flexion at the knee and sit on the table below her knee. Rest her foot on your shoulder or chest (depending on your size and the size of the leg). In this position you can use the hands or the forearms to work on the gastrocnemius and soleus muscles

(Photo 40). You can also stand at the side of the table to work on the client's posterior leg. Flex your knee and place it on the table just below the client's knee. Rest the client's foot on your thigh above your knee. In this position, you can comfortably address the leg with your hands or forearms.

Be aware that if your client is short and you have a long table, you will have to lean forward to reach his feet from the end of the table. You will be at a biomechanical disadvantage that is stressful to your body. In this case, ask your client to move down on the table until her feet are close to the end and within easy reach. Do not work on the feet from the side, because you will invariably end up deviating your wrists as you work (Photo 41) or twisting your trunk.

Some therapists like to sit down to work on the feet or the head/neck. For you to massage comfortably and safely while sitting, you will have to carefully adjust the height of the chair, the client, and/or the table. The chair must be high enough to allow you to use your upper body weight to create pressure (or the client must be lowered to accomplish the same objective). It must also be low enough that you can place your feet flat on the floor as you work, to create a stable base for the work of your upper body. Ideally, you should use a chair that is on rollers so you can reposition yourself easily.

Seated

Another comfortable way for the therapist to work is with the client seated in an on-site chair. It is easy for the therapist to remain upright at all times, and she can use her entire body to create his motions. You can use your forearms and elbows extensively with the client in this position, particularly on the back and shoulders. The arms and hands are quite accessible, since they are supported by a platform in front of client. The head can be easily

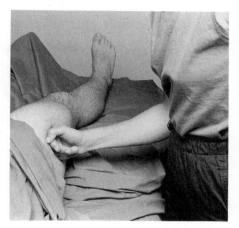

Photo 39

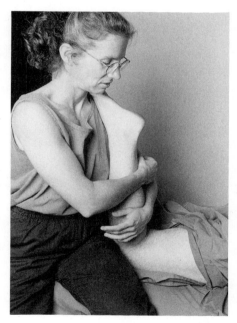

Photo 40

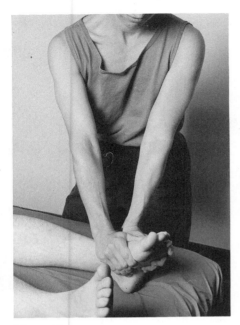

Photo 41

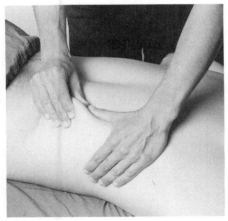

Photo 42

approached from the front as well.

One of the few disadvantages of seated massage is the tendency of the therapist to hyperextend, hyperflex and ulnar deviate the wrists when working on the back. Those who do seated massage need to be particularly careful about keeping the wrists straight as they massage.

Using Positioning Aids To Make Your Work Easier

There are several products that are now available to massage therapists that can maximize both the client's comfort and your own. These supports allow you to adjust the client's position to give you better access to whatever part of her body you want to massage. They also provide extra support and cushioning for clients with special needs, including pregnant women and persons with low back pain. The "Pivot Therapy Set" and the "bodyCushion™" are two such support systems that you can try.

Techniques to Approach with Caution (or Avoid Altogether)

Open C, Closed C

This petrissage technique uses the hands in the shape of a "C" to lift and push tissue between them. The palm and the ulnar side of the hand push the tissue and the thumb and index finger move together to grip and squeeze the tissue (Photo 42). This repetitive gripping and squeezing are stressful to the thumbs, hands and forearm flexors. To make this technique easier on your upper extremity, let the motion that creates the stroke come from the shoulders. Do just the pushing part of the stroke, not the gripping part, so you can rest your thumbs. If you find the technique uncomfortable, stop doing it altogether. Remember that there are other ways of doing petrissage, including the Lomi Lomi technique of circling with the forearm (see above).

Lifting

Many massage techniques require the therapist to lift a part of the client's body. Stop and think before you lift any body part. Consider the possible weight and whether you are strong enough to lift it. Take into consideration as well whether you will be lifting momentarily, or whether you will be holding the body part suspended for any amount of time. This awareness can keep you from being injured.

If you are already having symptoms or are injured, you will have no choice but to stop lifting altogether to prevent reinjury. There is nothing wrong with asking your client to lift his leg momentarily so you can pass the sheet under it to drape him, as long as he has no back or leg complaints. Asking a client to participate in his own treatment actually can empower him and make him feel more involved. Some treatment techniques call for the client to do active movement during the massage. In most cases, there are alternatives to lifting heavy body parts. Here are several examples:

Alternatives to Lifting and Holding Client's Head

Instead of holding your client's head while you work on the posterior neck, lift it for a moment and then place a folded towel under the top of his head to elevate it. To avoid lifting the head at all, roll the client's head to one side and place a small folded towel underneath the top of the head. Roll her head to the other side so it rolls onto the towel. The top of her head will now be supported and a space created for your hands to slip under her neck (Photo 43). You can also choose not to work on the neck in supine position at all. Do this work in side-lying or prone position.

Alternatives to Lifting Client's Torso

Doing back work with the client in supine position is extremely stressful. Some massage therapists do a paraspinal technique in this position that feels great for the client, but can easily injure the therapist. Standing or sitting at the client's head, the therapist forces his hands

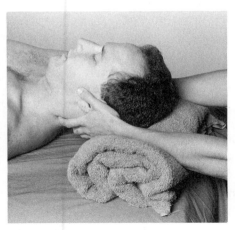

Photo 43

under the client's torso as far as he can reach. He then pushes up into the paraspinal muscles with his fingertips as he pulls his hands toward the client's head to achieve a long, deep friction of these muscles. While he is doing this technique, the fingertips are supporting much of the weight of the client's torso, placing tremendous stress on the therapist's fingers and forearm flexors. The technique is stressful enough if the therapist pulls back with his entire body. If he uses her arms alone to pull, the stress is greatly increased.

Only a very strong massage therapist could successfully do this technique without hurting herself. Since the back muscles can be addressed easily in either prone or sidelying position, there is no reason at all to do this technique.

Alternatives to Lifting Client's Shoulder

With the client prone, therapists often will lift the shoulder either to access the front of the shoulder, to manipulate the shoulder joint or to make the scapula wing out to access its medial border. The result of extended lifting is often shaking hands that are straining from the weight. Again, unless you are very strong, do not lift the shoulder or hold it up for any amount of time. Remember that shoulder work, both massage and mobilization, can be done quite nicely in both supine and sidelying positions. If you feel you want to work on the shoulder with your client prone, take a bolster or small pillow and place it under the client's shoulder to support it as you work. Ask the client to roll slightly to the other side to allow you to position the pillow -- do not lift the shoulder! Using a bolster or pillow can often take the place of lifting and suspending parts of the body. The medial border of the scapula can be made more prominent by placing the client's hand behind her low back instead of lifting the shoulder.

Supine neck work

Massage therapists are often taught to work on the posterior neck muscles while sitting at the client's head. The therapist places his hands on either side of the cervical spine to massage the muscles. In this position, the therapist's hands tend to go into excessive ulnar deviation. Make sure you keep your wrists straight when working on this area to avoid wrist injury.

Suboccipital release is another popular massage technique also done with the client supine. The therapist lifts the head, placing it on her curled fingertips. The weight of the head creates the direct pressure on the suboccipital muscles. It also strains the therapist's forearm flexor muscles. The suboccipital muscles can be approached with the client in sidelying or prone position. If you choose to continue to work on these muscles with the client supine, make a loose fist with both hands and roll the

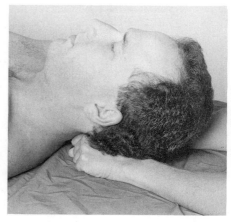

Photo 44

client's head onto your metacarpophalangeal knuckles (Photo 44). Do not press upward with your hands. Encourage the client to let her head sink down onto your knuckles, and allow the weight of the head to provide the pressure.

Tractioning

To safely provide traction to the leg, grab the client's ankle and heel, keeping the wrists straight. Stabilize your scapulas, keep your arms straight, and lean back to allow your body weight to create the traction. Do not lift the leg! Let it slide along the table as you pull back with your body. Again, this will be easier to do with a hydraulic table. The head and the arm can be put in traction in the same manner.

Effleurage of Legs with Deviated Hands

This technique involves long strokes with the palms on the anterior and posterior legs and thighs. To create the stroke, you must put one hand into ulnar deviation and the other hand into radial deviation (Photo 45). Instead, keep your wrists straight as you massage the lower extremity. Better yet, use your forearms to work on the legs and thighs.

Tapotement

Keep your upper body loose and your hands soft as you apply fast tapotement strokes to avoid any tension that could contribute to injury. Make sure the shoulders remain level and the scapulas stable as you do your tapotement technique.

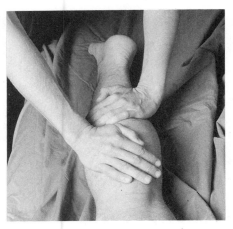

Photo 45

Using Other Modalities In Your Massages

There are many modalities that can be used during a massage session that do not require using your hands. Many of these can replace hand/arm-intensive techniques altogether. Hydrotherapy, heat application, aromatherapy, and joint mobilization are just a few modalities that can be used to create overall relaxation and treat specific complaints. These methods are much easier on your body than manual massage techniques that use pressure, and are often just as effective.

For example, you may spend ten minutes manually massaging a client's shoulders in an attempt to make hypertonic muscles more pliable. You can spare your body the physical work of softening these muscles by applying moist heat for the same amount of time. You may be able to relieve a client's headache by administering a warm, lavender-scented foot bath, placing a cold pack on his forehead, and laying a warm, moist compress on his neck. Gently massaging scented oils or topical analgesics like Tiger Balm® into the skin in areas of tension or pain can be both soothing and therapeutic.

Take some time in your massage session to teach your client some mobilizations and stretches that he can do at home. Watch him do these in front of you to make sure that his form is correct. Spending five or ten minutes of a massage working with the client in this manner cuts down on stress to your body, and gives your client an opportunity to participate in his own healing.

Continue to experiment with modifying your technique and finding alternative modalities that can reduce stress to your body. If some of the alternate techniques suggested here do not feel comfortable for you, try a different approach. The process of experimentation can be as important as the resulting new techniques. With every experiment, you will develop greater body awareness. After a while, you will know your body and how it responds to massage so thoroughly that avoiding injury will become a much easier task.

7

Exercises and Stretches for the Massage Athelete

To have a long, healthy career in massage, you need to become a massage "athlete." Like an athlete, you must build and maintain strength and endurance, and counteract muscular tension resulting from the physical activity of your work. Like an athlete, you should count on working out at least three times a week, using a combination of strengthening exercises, stretches, and aerobic conditioning. The exercises described in this chapter offer a good, basic program of strengthening and stretching specially designed for massage therapists with the help of two very experienced physical therapists.

You may add to this basic program any exercises that address the back, the abdominals, and the legs. Do not add more hand or arm exercises that are repetitive in nature. Most aerobic activities are fine for massage therapists, as long as they do not tax the arms in any significant way. Swimming, running, walking, hiking, dancing, and low-impact aerobics classes are good, safe choices. Walking is great exercise, especially for persons who have not previously been physically active. Sports like tennis, squash, racquetball, and volleyball should be avoided since they put strain on the arms. Even bicycling can be hard on the hands and wrists, since they must absorb vibration and shock from the handlebars. Use common sense in your exercise program to avoid further trauma to your already overused hands.

The stretches and exercises below are designed to deal with the consequences of doing massage work. Massage therapists spend a great deal of their time doing strenuous work with their arms in front of their bodies. As a result, the front of the body gets overworked and tight, while the back gets overstretched and weak. This imbalance between the anterior and posterior musculature makes it impossible for the muscles to exert an even pull on the upper extremity to help with its work. The upper extremity ends up being overused to compensate for the lack of proximal support and strength.

You can resolve this imbalance by stretching the front of the body, which is tight from overuse, and strengthening the back of the body, which is weak from underuse. The operative principle is to counteract the forces that are creating the problem. For example, many people have low back problems because they bend forward in their everday lives (sitting at a desk, picking things up) much more than they bend backward. The spine extensors become weak from disuse, which makes them prone to injury. Back extension exercises are often prescribed for low back pain to create balance between the flexors and the extensors.

For these exercises and stretches to be safe and effective, they must be done in correct form. Just as alignment is important in your massage movements to prevent injury, it is also important to keep in mind as you stretch and exercise, so that these activities do not cause or aggravate injury.

Stretching

Stretching will help get your muscles ready to work before you massage, and will help them relax after you massage. It will encourage good circulation into the muscle and tendon tissue, making the tissues more pliable and less likely to tear. Stretch frequently throughout the day, whenever you feel stiff or fatigued, especially after any period of inactivity. Schedule time to stretch before and after each massage you give to refresh yourself (and keep yourself from doing back-to-back massages).

These stretches are designed to increase the flow of blood, energy, breath, and nerve impulses to the upper extremity by stretching the muscles of the neck, shoulder, and chest, as well as those of the arm itself. They will also increase circulation to the proximal muscles, so they will be ready to support the use of your arms.

All of these stretches should be done within an active, pain-free range of motion. Go into each stretch slowly so you have time to pay attention to the sensation you feel. Stretch to the point where you *begin* to feel a good stretch, not the point where you feel the muscle is just about to tear. Do not try to force the stretch past this point. Do not bounce. If you feel discomfort, you have stretched too much: back off a bit. If you feel pain, you may be injured. Discontinue stretching until you see a doctor.

Do each stretch once, holding the position for thirty seconds to one minute. Make sure you continue to *breathe normally* throughout the entire stretch to encourage your muscles to relax.

Wrist Flexor Stretch

Sit at a desk or table that is at a comfortable height. With your arms in front of you, bend them at the elbow and place your palms against the edge of the table with the fingers pointing up. Relax the hands and forearms. Keeping the forearms straight and parallel to each other, lean slowly against the table with your palms until you begin to feel a stretch. Breathe!

Wrist Extensor Stretch

Same position as above, but place the backs of the hands against the edge of the table with the fingers pointing toward the floor. Keeping the forearms straight and parallel to each other, lean slowly against the table with the backs of your hands until you begin to feel a stretch. Breathe!

Neck Stretches

Sit in a chair, with your feet flat on the floor, your low back supported by a pillow, your hands in your lap. Raise your chest so that your head and shoulders fall naturally into a neutral position. After each stretch you will return to a neutral head position, looking straight forward with your chin level. The neck is delicate and can be easily injured, so do each of these stretches in a slow, controlled manner.

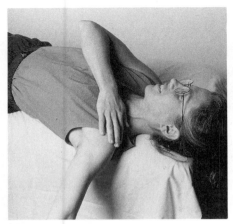

Photo 46

Ear to Shoulder: Keeping the shoulders level and facing squarely forward, bend your head to the left so the left ear moves toward the left shoulder. Hold where you begin to feel the stretch. Breathe! Return head slowly to neutral, then do the same motion to the right.

Look Over Your Shoulder: Keeping the shoulders level and facing squarely forward, turn you head to the left as if you were trying to look over your left shoulder. Keep your chin on the same plane as you rotate; do not let your chin lift up. Hold where you begin to feel the stretch. Breathe! Return head slowly to neutral, then do the same motion to the right.

Chin to Chest: Tuck your chin, then slowly move your chin down toward your chest until you feel the stretch. Hold there and breathe! Return head slowly to neutral.

Note: Do not do head/neck "rolls" (circumduction of the head). They are too stressful to the neck.

Pectoralis Major Stretch

Lie down supine in a diagonal on your massage table, so the right side of the upper body is close to the edge of the table and your lower body and legs are more securely centered on the table (so you don't roll off). Hang your left arm and shoulder off the side of the table with your palm facing up, and place your right hand on the front of your left shoulder (Photo 46). Relax the right shoulder and arm, so the weight of the arm can stretch the pectoralis major muscle. Breathe! With your left hand, make sure the right shoulder does not move forward. Keep the arm straight out at a 90° angle to your body. Repeat with the left arm.

Lattisimus Dorsi Stretch

Lie supine with your body centered on your massage table and your arms straight by your sides. Bend your knees to flatten your low back against the table. With your thumb pointing up, raise your right arm straight up and over your head. The thumb will now be pointing at the floor (Photo 47). Keep your arm straight (do not bend your elbow). Make sure you keep your low back flat against the table as you lift the arm. Hold your position when you feel the stretch in the lats. Breathe! Lower your arm and repeat with the other arm.

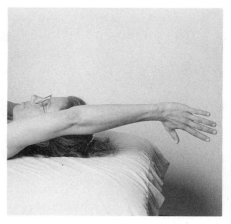

Photo 47

Pronation Self-Mobilization and Stretch

People who do hand-intensive work tend to have reduced ROM in pronation. The muscles of the forearm become so overused and tense that they restrict movement of the radius and ulna at the proximal and distal radioulnar joints. People with this limited ROM compensate at the wrist by forcing the carpal bones into excessive pronation. The carpal bones give a bit to allow this to happen. This extra motion puts pressure on the carpal bones and changes the size of the carpal tunnel (contributing to CTS). Compensation happens also at the shoulder. To achieve greater ROM in pronation, people abduct and internal rotate the shoulders, bringing the elbows out to the side. This motion encourages the hands to go into ulnar deviation, another harmful posture for massage work (see Photo 29, Chapter 6).

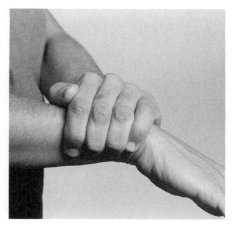

Photo 48

Do the following stretch/mobilization to counteract the stress put on the wrist and the hand by excessive pronation of the forearms. Tuck your right elbow against your side. Turn your palm down, and relax the wrist and the hand to avoid straining them. Place your left palm across the top of your forearm proximal to the radiostyloid process and wrap your fingers around the ulna (Photo 48). Do not wrap the fingers around too far, or you may put pressure on the carpal tunnel! Pull the ulna superiorly and push the radius inferiorly at the same time, thus moving the bones further into pronation. Hold this position for 30 seconds to one minute to stretch tight forearm muscles, or do a series of short repetitions as a mobilization to loosen up the proximal and distal radioulnar joints. Repeat with right arm.

You may do other stretches in addition to these, as long as you avoid stretching the upper back. This area is already stretched out, and should not be stretched further. Stretching the low back and legs, especially the hamstrings, will relieve the tension that can develop in those areas as a result of doing massage. They will also help get your blood circulating throughout your entire body.

Routine Strengthening Exercises

The massage "athlete" needs to train and stay in shape to keep up with the demands of a massage career. To do that, you will need to make room in your life for regular exercise. It is best to start getting in shape even before you start studying massage, and certainly during the time you are a student. However, it is never too late to start developing strength and stamina. As long as you are healthy and not experiencing any signs or symptoms of injury, you can start doing the following conditioning exercises. They will help you develop proximal strength to stabilize your scapulas and provide support for the work of your arms. Building distal arm strength is also important, so that your arms and hands will be able to withstand the pressure you place on them when you massage. If any of these exercises cause any pain or discomfort, back off on the intensity or stop doing the exercise completely. These are meant to be challenging; they should not be painful.

Note: If you are over the age of 45 or have a history of major or chronic illness, consult your physician before beginning any exercise program.

If you are already experiencing any symptom of injury, DO NOT DO THESE EXERCISES. You need to see a health care practitioner trained in rehabilitation (most likely a physical or occupational therapist) who can prescribe an exercise program for you once your acute symptoms have subsided. Once you have completely healed, you can review these exercises with the practitioner you have been seeing to determine whether they are appropriate for you to start doing to stay in shape.

Proximal Strength Exercises

These exercises will help you counteract the forward shoulder and head posture that massage therapists tend to work in by strengthening the large muscles of the back and chest. Do this group of exercises three times per week.

Wall Arm Lifts - Emphasizes muscle balance

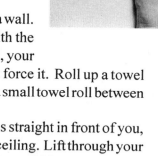

Muscles Used: Lower abdominals, cervical retraction muscles, lower and middle trapezius, thoracic paraspinals (extensors), rhomboids.

Position: Stand with your back against a wall. Your head should also be against the wall with the chin level. (If you are very round-shouldered, your

Photo 49

head will not go back against the wall - don't force it. Roll up a towel and place it behind your head instead.) Place a small towel roll between the wall and your lower back.

Exercise 1: 180° Flexion. Lift both arms straight in front of you, keeping arms straight and thumbs toward the ceiling. Lift through your entire shoulder ROM, up over your head to the wall if you can. Make sure your scapulas stay fairly flat against the wall as you lift your arms. Your head should remain against the wall, and your chin should stay level. Do not arch your back; rather, use your lower abdominals to keep your lower back against the towel roll. Repeat 10-15 times.

Exercise 2: "V" for Victory!. Put your hands up to the sides of your head, like a traffic cop saying "stop." If it is comfortable, put your elbows against the wall (if it is not, don't do it). Keeping your scapulas fairly flat against the wall, lift your arms up into the shape of a "V," sliding your hands against the wall if you can (Photo 49). Finally, lift the arms until they are straight over your head with the hands touching each other. Repeat 10-15 times.

Shoulder Pullbacks - Strengthens the upper back muscles to keep the scapulas stable

Muscles Used: Rhomboids, lower and middle trapezius
Position: Get a stretchy band, either surgical tubing with handles or several giant rubber bands tied together. Anchor your stretchy band in a door at elbow height, and stretch it toward you while keeping it parallel to the floor.

Exercise: Keeping your arms absolutely straight, pull back evenly on the stretchy band by pinching your shoulder blades

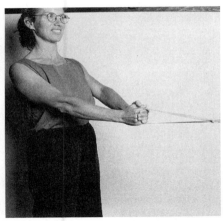

Photo 50

together (photo 50). Make sure that your head does not jut forward as you pull back, and that your shoulders remain level and do not lift. Hold for a few seconds, then let the stretchy band relax slowly and evenly.

Repetitions: Start at 5-10 for strengthening, work up to 30 for endurance.

Pull-Ups - Strengthens the upper back muscles to create scapular stabilization while also working the distal arm muscles.

Muscles Used: Middle and lower trapezius, rhomboids, wrist and finger flexors, biceps.

Position: Place a broom handle, stick or dowel between two surfaces of roughly the same height (two massage tables would be ideal, or your massage table adjusted to the height of a nearby table or desk). Leave enough room between the two surfaces for your body to fit. Sit down on the floor between the two surfaces with the stick above and slightly in front of you (about one foot). Place hands on top of stick, with fingers facing down. With your hands on top of the stick, you should be sitting with your back only halfway upright. Grasp the stick (not too tightly!) with straight arms (Photo 51).

Exercise: Keeping your buttocks on the floor, pull your upper body up and forward toward the stick by pinching your shoulder blades together. Allow your elbows to bend as you come up (Photo 52). Make sure you are not using your abdominal muscles to accomplish the movement - you want to work you upper back, not your abdominals! (Also be sure not to pull up with your arm muscles exclusively, which would put too much strain on them.) When your back is upright, hold for a few seconds, then slowly lower yourself back down into your original position.

Advanced version (buttocks lifts): Position is the same. Pinching your shoulder blades together, lift your upper body up and forward toward the stick. When your back has reached upright position, keep going until your butt lifts off the floor. Hold position for several seconds, then slowly lower yourself back down into your original position.

Repetitions: 5-10 to start, work up to 30

Wall Push-ups - Builds both chest and back muscles while also working distal arm muscles.

Muscles Used: Finger flexors, wrist flexors and extensors, pectoralis major, serratus anterior, triceps, trapezius as stabilizer.

Position: Stand about one foot from a wall, facing it. Place pads of fingers against the wall; your palms should not touch it. Elbows and hands should be shoulder-width apart.

Exercise: Lean forward against the wall, allowing elbows to move out to the sides (laterally), and keeping your wrists in neutral position. Make sure shoulders stay level. Use your fingertips to support your weight (about 1/3 of your total body weight) (Photo 53). Hold for several seconds, then push against wall with your fingertips to return body to upright position.

Advanced Version: Same position and moves, but stand farther away from wall.

Repetitions: 5-10 to start, work up to 30

Distal Strength Exercises

These exercises help strengthen the small muscles of the fingers, hand, wrist, and arm. Do them three times per week. For the exercises that use weights, be sure to start out with very light weights, one or two pounds. You can always increase the weight later, but you don't want to hurt yourself when you start out. If you are concerned about over-gripping the weight, you can use wrist cuff weights and concentrate on keeping your hands relaxed while working the other muscles.

Hand Squeezes - Builds strength in the intrinsic muscles of the hand

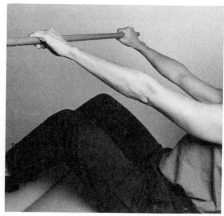

Photo 51

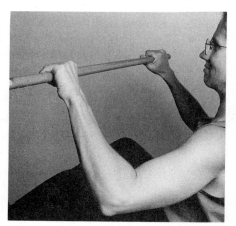

Photo 52

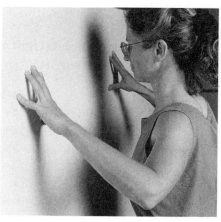

Photo 53

Get a variety of objects that you can squeeze in the palm of your hand: a tennis ball, some Power Putty, a gripper-exerciser, etc. Squeezing a variety of objects instead of just one will keep you from overworking or overusing any one set of muscles, which in itself could cause injury. Vary the size of the objects as well. Squeezing different sized objects will help you develop strength throughout the ROM of the finger flexors.

Exercise: Keeping the wrist neutral (neither flexed nor extended), take one of the objects and squeeze it with moderate strength 10-15 times. Work at a comfortable pace, slow enough to control the motion in and out. Make sure you completely relax the muscles between each repetition. Work both hands in the same way. The next time you do this exercise, use a different object. Keep alternating from session to session.

Open and Close Hands-Stabilizes and balances the musculature around the wrist joint.

This exercise is meant to train your movement pattern rather than to build strength or endurance.

Position: Put your hand out comfortably in front of you like you were going to shake hands with someone (thumb up). Concentrate on the wrist, which needs to remain absolutely stable and neutral.

Exercise: Open your hand slowly, keeping the wrist neutral at all times. Close the hand slowly to a loose fist, keeping the wrist neutral at all times. Open and close the hand 30 times, then do other hand.

Free-Weight Roll-Ups - Builds strength in the forearm flexors and extensors.

Overhand Position: Tie a one-pound weight to a stick, dowel or broom handle with some heavy string. Place your hands on top of stick, holding it in your hands with the palms down. Elbows should be bent 90°, hands shoulder-width apart. Try not to grip the stick too tightly as you do the exercise.

Exercise: Roll the stick toward you, so the string wraps around the side of the stick facing away from you (Photo 54). When the weight reaches the stick, roll the weight back down in the opposite direction. Repeat 10 times.

Underhand Position: Place the stick on top of your hands with the palms facing up. Elbows should be bent 90°, hands shoulder-width apart.

Exercise: Roll the stick toward you, so the string wraps around the outside of the stick. When the weight reaches the stick, roll the weight back down in the opposite direction. Repeat 10 times.

Increase weight slowly and gradually as your strength increases.

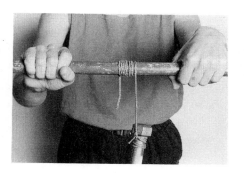

Photo 54

Biceps Curls - Builds strength in biceps muscles.

Position: Do this exercise standing with your back against a wall.

Exercise: Start with a one or two pound weight. Hold the weight in your right hand, palm up. Begin with your arm at your side with the elbow straight. Keep your scapulas fairly flat against the wall as you move. Place your left hand on the front of your right shoulder to make sure the shoulder does not roll forward as you lift the weight. Bring the weight forward until it almost touches your shoulder. Hold for a few seconds, then lower the arm to starting position. Control the motion up and down so it is somewhat slow and very even. Be sure not to arch your low back as you move the arm up or down. Repeat 10-15 times. Do same exercise with left arm.

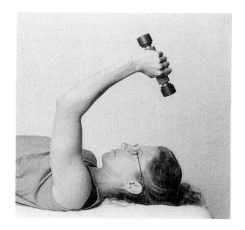

Photo 55

Increase weight slowly and gradually as your strength increases.

Triceps Dips - Builds strength in triceps muscles.

Position: Lie down on your back on a bench or massage table with bent knees. This position keeps the neck supported so it does not get strained. Make sure you do not lift your chin or arch your neck during

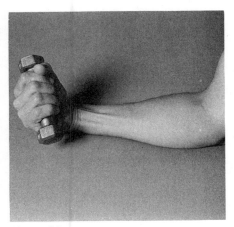

Photo 56

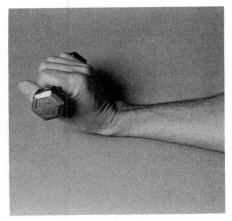

Photo 57

the exercise. Hold a one or two pound weight in your right hand, thumb pointing toward your head. Raise your arm so it is straight over your chest, at a 90° angle to your body. Be sure to keep your low back pressed into the bench as you move.

Exercise: Dip weight down toward your shoulder, bending the elbow but keeping the tip of the elbow pointing straight up (Photo 55). Straighten arm again and hold for several seconds. Repeat 10-15 times. Make sure motions are slow and controlled. Do same exercise with left arm.

Wrist Curls - Strengthens muscles working on the wrist joint

(Note: Massage therapists use their wrist flexors a great deal in their work, and the wrist extensors tend to get weak. It is very important to strengthen the wrist extensors to balance the forces acting on the wrist. Therefore, be sure to do all three sets of exercises.)

<u>Wrist Flexion Position:</u> Sit at a table or desk that is not too high. Lay right elbow, forearm and hand down on the table in front of you. Table should be a height which allows you to rest your forearm on it without having to raise your upper arm or shoulder. Hold a one pound weight in your right hand with palm facing up.

Exercise: Making sure that the forearm stays on the table, flex the wrist. Hold for several seconds, then let the hand go back down to table (Photo 56). Repeat 10-15 times. Be sure to completely relax the muscles between each repetition.

<u>Wrist Extension Position:</u> Turn arm over so palm is facing down.

Exercise: Making sure that the forearm stays on the table, extend the wrist. Hold for several seconds, then let the hand go back down to the table (Photo 57). Repeat 10-15 times. Be sure to completely relax the muscles between each repetition.

<u>Wrist Radial Deviation Position:</u> Rest right elbow on the table, with forearm vertical on table. Hold weight in hand with palm facing away from body.

Exercise: Radially deviate the hand at the wrist (Photo 58). Hold for several seconds, then return hand to neutral. Repeat 10-15 times. Be sure to completely relax the muscles between each repetition.

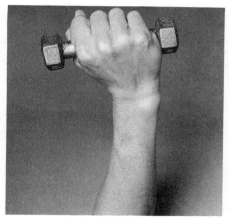

Photo 58

Breathing Exercises

Learning to breathe deeply and regularly will help you counteract tension as you work. It's also great for your health!

Finding the Bottom of the Breath

The point of this exercise is to notice how the breath works when tension is removed, so you can develop a natural, conscious way of breathing fully and deeply. Think about letting the breath happen naturally instead of forcing yourself to breath in any special way.

Sit in a chair, close your eyes and relax. Take a breath and exhale naturally through your mouth - don't force the breath out. Keep exhaling until your breath is used up. Relax, and wait. If you think of the breath as a long, vertical oval, this is the "bottom" of your breath. Wait until you can clearly feel the impulse to breathe. It is not necessary to wait until you are desperate for air, just until you can identify that your body wants to breathe. Try to notice where in your body the impulse to breathe originates. Most persons feel the impulse originating in the abdomen or below the rib cage. Take a normal breath in through your nose. Notice when the breath crests at the "top" and turns into an exhale. Exhale through your mouth again. Keep exhaling until your breath is used up, and wait again at the bottom. Repeat as many times as is comfortable. If you do this exercise correctly, you should not hyperventilate or feel at all dizzy.

Lateral Rib Expansion

When you breathe shallowly, the diaphragm cannot do as much of the work of breathing as it should. Underutilizing the diaphragm causes you to overutilize the secondary muscles of respiration, including the scalenes, the upper trapezii, and the intrinsic neck muscles. These muscles can become hypertonic from overuse, making you more susceptible to thoracic outlet syndrome. The diaphragm becomes weak from underuse. Expanding the ribs laterally as you breath develops and strengthens the diaphragm. A stronger diaphragm will participate more fully in breathing.

Stand in front of a full-length mirror. As you breathe in deeply, concentrate on expanding your rib cage laterally. You should be able to see the ribs clearly expand out to the sides. Exhale. It may take some practice before you can isolate your breathing in this way. Your goal is make the rib cage expand laterally by two to three inches. You can take a soft tape measure and measure the girth of your ribs before and after inhalation to judge your progress.

Yoga Breathing Exercises

These exercises emphasize deep, full, conscious breathing. They will make a good addition to your repertoire. If you do not know any of these exercises, there are many good books available that offer a number of different Yoga breathing exercises from which to choose.

Suggested Workout Routine

You can combine all of the stretches and exercises in this chapter into an exercise routine that can be done individually or as a class in 1/2 hour to 45 minutes:

1. Warm ups (stretches, breathing, and jogging in place or other light aerobics)

2. Proximal muscle exercises in this book

3. Distal muscle exercises in this book

5. Cool down (stretches, breathing, guided imagery to create a feeling of health and well-being).

Work on Your Body Alignment

Movement-centered disciplines like Feldenkrais and Alexander Technique teach students how to move their body in less stressful ways to encourage overall health. The emphasis is on moving the body as one unit, and using physical properties like weight and joint alignment to help create movement. Movement training can be extremely helpful for massage therapists, particularly those who have not had experience with dance, sports or other disciplines that teach coordination, grace and ease of movement.

As you become stronger and more at ease with your body, you should notice a difference in the way you do massage. Your strokes should become more even and controlled. You should have greater energy and endurance, so that you feel less tired at the end of a work day. You may feel generally more competent, like you can handle almost any situation that presents itself as you work. A feeling of physical strength and grace can be very empowering, and can add a new dimension to your massage work, both emotionally and physically.

Taking the time to exercise and stretch at least three times each week also gives you a wonderful opportunity to develop your body awareness. Your workout sessions are a time to get in touch with your body, to see how it responds to limited amounts of stress in a controlled situation. Focus on your physical reactions to the stretches and exercises you do. Notice which parts of your body move easily, and which feel more restricted. Note which muscle groups are tight and which are looser, which are weak and which are stronger. After you have been working out for a while, you will become intimately familiar with your own body. Using this increased body awareness as you massage will enable you to notice your reactions to the physical work you are doing, and to empathize with your clients' response to your massaging.

8

Treatment

Inevitably, some massage therapists will end up getting injured. The ups and downs of life can interfere with even the best intentions and most careful surveillance of lifestyle and work habits. Becoming injured is not shameful. It is merely an occupational hazard.

If you should become injured as a result of your massage work, there are a number of options available to you to resolve your injury. Good, effective treatments are out there; it is just a matter of knowing how to find them. Finding the best possible treatments will make your recovery faster and easier.

To properly treat your symptoms, three things must be determined:

1. What is the injury process? (diagnosis);
2. What triggered the injury? (onset); and
3. What is the extent of the injury (severity).

Many massage therapists try to make these determinations themselves, with varying levels of success. It takes perspective and objectivity to evaluate a medical condition accurately. Even physicians are told not to self-diagnose or self-treat. Massage therapists also do not have the training to make diagnoses. Still, many therapists try to self-treat and see what kind of results they can get before seeking help from other health practitioners. This approach is certainly better than totally ignoring the problem, the route too many people take.

The impetus to self-treat can come from a desire to stay self-reliant, which is understandable. The urge to self-treat can also come from shame, not wanting to tell anyone you are injured because you see it is a failure of sorts. It makes people feel vulnerable to say they have a problem and ask others for help. You may be afraid that the doctor will confirm that you are indeed injured, and then you will be forced to take the injury seriously instead of continuing to fool yourself that it will go away on its own. Financial considerations also may enter into your decision to self-treat. Medical care can be costly, especially if you are not insured. If you must decrease your workload to allow your injury to heal, your financial health may suffer as well. You may want to self-treat because it seems like the easiest and quickest way to make this annoying and upsetting problem go away quickly.

Despite all of these arguments, the wisest course of action is to see a physician as early in the injury process as you can. If you have been experiencing symptoms for longer than a few weeks, it is unlikely that self-treatment will have much effect. It can also waste valuable time while your injury worsens. If you have just begun to feel mild symptoms and you are intent on self-treatment, set a time limit and monitor your symptoms carefully. Try your "treatment of choice" for a week or two, whether it be massage, hydrotherapy, over-the-counter anti-inflammatory medication, acupuncture, rest, or any combination thereof. If by the end of that period of time your symptoms are not considerably better, see a doctor. Certainly if the symptoms get worse during that time, or if new symptoms appear, go to a doctor right away. A minor injury that could have been treated easily can quickly turn into a complicated, chronic injury that takes a long time to resolve and affects your ability to continue massaging. It can cripple your hands and ruin your quality of life. It cannot be emphasized enough how important it is to catch and treat these injuries early.

How Do I Know When To See A Physician?

There are a number of criteria you can use to determine if it is time for you to see a physician. You should certainly see a doctor if you are experiencing severe pain, particularly if the pain persists longer than three or four days. Follow this guideline regardless of whether the pain is constant or intermittent. Even occasional severe pain should be reported to a doctor and followed carefully. Swelling is a sure sign of injury. If you see any swelling at or near the injury site, consult a physician.

Some signs of injury are less obvious than pain or swelling. Many massage therapists report that they first became concerned that they might be injured when they began to have trouble performing ordinary, day-to-day activities. If you feel pain or discomfort when opening a door, brushing your teeth or hair, or writing, you should schedule an appointment with a physician.

Diagnosis – A Necessary First Step

Getting a diagnosis is a necessary prelude to treatment. At this time, only medical doctors (M.D.'s) and osteopaths (D.O.'s) are allowed by law to diagnose throughout the United States; naturopathic doctors (N.D.'s) are licensed to diagnose as well in some states. Usually your doctor will be able to give you at least a preliminary diagnosis that can be used to start you on a treatment plan. Sometimes it takes more visits and more tests such as X-rays and blood work before she can figure out exactly what is causing your symptoms and how to treat them properly. Often physical therapists can provide additional information to the physician and make the true diagnosis more apparent. There is much that medical science does not yet understand about repetitive stress injuries, and there may be a number of injury processes going on at the same time which can present a confusing, overlapping array of symptoms. You doctor will, however, be able to rule out a number of other health problems, including systemic disease, that may be a contributing factor to, or even the primary cause of, your symptoms.

Selecting a Doctor

Finding a good doctor to treat your injury is critical. Unfortunately, many massage therapists report that this can be a frustrating experience. Some therapists end up not going to a doctor at all because they have no idea whom to choose and by what criteria. A number of therapists who have seen doctors complain that these physicians were unresponsive or insensitive to them, did not have much to offer in the way of effective treatment methods, or misdiagnosed and subsequently mistreated them.

Some offered unusual or extreme treatments, like putting an injured arm in a cast for six weeks to "rest" the injury. Others told them to simply stop doing massage, which for some therapists was economically impossible. Such experiences cause massage therapists to lose faith in allopathic medicine.

There are, however, a good number of physicians who do know how to diagnose and treat repetitive stress injuries and do it quite well. They have acquired the extra training needed to make accurate diagnoses, and have developed the sensitivity and compassion to work with you effectively to get you healthy again. They can also be humble enough to know when they reach the limits of what they can do and refer you to specialists or physical therapists (whom doctors are beginning to accept as important colleagues in treating repetitive stress injuries). The key to finding a good doctor is knowing what to look for and not being afraid to ask for what you need.

You will want to see a physician who is well versed and completely up-to-date on RSI's and the best treatments for them. Your primary care physician is your first resource, and can make a preliminary diagnosis of your condition. If your case is complicated or difficult to diagnose, the primary care physician may refer you to a specialist. Sports medicine doctors, orthopedists who specialize in injury brought on by intense physical activity, now treat many occupation-caused RSI's as well, as do physiatrists (specialists in physical medicine and rehabilitation). If you do not have a primary care doctor, ask your teachers or a professional massage therapist that you trust if they know of a good doctor who is skilled at treating RSI's. You can also get referrals from hospitals, many of which now have occupational, physical medicine and/or sports medicine departments.

At some point in your treatment you may be referred to a hand specialist. These doctors are usually surgeons specializing in hand disorders. Keep in mind, though, that the more specialized the doctor, the more narrow her vision is likely to be in searching for a diagnosis. She may tend to look at the hand alone and may not take the rest of the upper extremity into consideration to find causes of symptoms. As you saw in Chapter 4, pain in the hand can be the result of an injury anywhere in the arm, shoulder, or neck. Looking at the hand by itself does not provide a big enough picture to make a good diagnosis. Specialists who are surgeons may tend to recommend surgery as the main feature of treatment. A good hand specialist will mention surgery as one option among others, and will tell you the pros and cons of any proposed surgical procedure. Unless you have an advanced case of a nerve impingement injury like carpal tunnel syndrome, where permanent damage to the nerve is a distinct possibility, surgery can usually wait until other treatments have been tried.

Once you find a doctor with the right qualities, you will want to see if he asks the right questions and listens attentively to your responses. He should want to know much more about the injury than the just where it hurts and how long it has been a problem. He will need to take a full medical history, including a history of past injuries and illnesses, the treatments you have tried so far for this problem (what worked/didn't work), and what medications you are taking. He may run some blood tests to rule out illnesses such as rheumatoid arthritis that could be causing or contributing to the symptoms. There are additional tests that can give your doctor more information about your injury, including nerve conduction velocity (NCV) and arthroscopy. Some of these tests are quite simple; others are invasive, painful and expensive. Ask your doctor if the results of the test will change the way he treats the injury. If not, there may be no reason to do the test. Having a $600 NCV test done for a mild case of CTS may confirm that you do indeed have a mild case of CTS, but the treatment will be the same regardless. You might as well spare yourself the discomfort and expense of the test.

In addition to a medical history, your physician should want to know all about your life as a massage therapist: how many massages you do in a day, in a week; how long you have been doing massage; what techniques make the symptoms worse; and what kind of work environment you have (home studio, medical office, massage clinic, etc.). Questions about your lifestyle - eating, sleeping and exercise habits, tobacco and alcohol/drug use, etc. - are also appropriate and can help your doctor get a better picture of your overall health. After obtaining all of this information, she will do a complete examination of the affected areas, and also evaluate your overall posture and stance. A good doctor for repetitive stress injuries will want to look for possible proximal pathology that may be contributing to or causing your injury. If your wrist hurts and your doctor looks only at your wrist, you need to suggest that she look at your neck and shoulder as well. If she balks at this idea, get another doctor.

After arriving at a diagnosis, you doctor should work out a treatment plan with you that includes short-term symptom relief, rehabilitation of the injury, and changes in your massage work that will keep you from getting reinjured while you are healing. If your injury is very mild, you may be able to keep doing massage while you are in treatment as long as you figure out what caused the injury and stop doing it. Otherwise, your doctor will likely recommend that you curtail your workload or take time off from doing massage for a while. How long that will be will depend on the extent of your injury. If you have been referred to a physical, occupational, or massage therapist, sometimes he will be the one to work with you on changing your work habits instead of the physician.

If you become dissatisfied with the way your doctor is handling your case, it is always best to explain to her that you are not satisfied with her approach and would like her to do A, B, and C. Then give her a chance to respond. If she does not do many of the things mentioned above, if you feel she really doesn't listen to you, or if you just still feel uncomfortable with her after the second or third visit, move on. Remember that it is your prerogative to say "Thank you, but no thanks" and try a different doctor. You may also wish to obtain a second opinion to get another perspective on your condition.

Remember also that you share in the responsibility for your treatment with your physician. No doctor can help you if you don't follow his advice, or if you withhold information from him, or if you self-treat along with his treatments and don't coordinate that treatment with his treatment. Your physician is your ally in resolving your injury, not a miracle-worker who will magically make everything better. Working with your doctor on equal footing will empower you and facilitate proper treatment of your condition.

Physical Therapy and Occupational Therapy

Physicians often refer patients with RSI's to physical or occupational therapists for rehabilitation. Physical therapists concentrate on helping you develop good posture and regain strength and mobility.

Occupational therapists retrain patients to work and function in a manner that will prevent injury and reinjury. They also create custom-made splints to enable patients to continue to use their arms in their daily lives. Both PT's and OT's are trained to administer treatments that are effective for RSI's, including hydrotherapy, ultrasound, myofascial release and other types of soft tissue massage, strengthening exercises, and passive joint mobilization. You will see a PT or OT on a regular basis, often one to four times per week. They can be very helpful not only in delivering treatment, but also in encouraging and reassuring you as you heal and recover from your injury. Since you see them often, you can develop a strong relationship with your PT or OT, and they can become your "cheerleader," an ally in your recovery. For this reason it is important to find a PT or OT with whom you feel comfortable, someone in whom you can put your trust. If you don't feel a good rapport with the first PT or OT you see, you can ask your physician to recommend someone else. You may also wish to call several PT's and OT's to find one that specializes in manual therapy.

Finding Out What Caused the Injury

To properly treat the injury, you must determine what caused it. RSI's are usually caused by a combination of improper technique (awkward positioning especially) and pre-existing characteristics of the therapist, and some change in workload or work habits. A physician knowledgeable about RSI's can be helpful in making this determination by inquiring into your work and lifestyle and evaluating any inherent factors that increased your risk for injury. It would be wise also to consult with an experienced massage therapist or physical therapist who can watch you do a massage. These practitioners have more experience than physicians with hands-on work, and should be able to evaluate your technique and body mechanics. They can point out motions and positions that may be putting too much strain on the injured body part, and suggest alternative moves that are less stressful to your upper extremity. They should also evaluate your standing and sitting posture, as well as certain movement patterns which may be contributing to injury. If your posture is implicated in your injury, your PT or OT can prescribe exercise, stretching, and posture/movement re-education to correct it as part of your treatment.

Specific Treatments to Resolve Injury

The primary goals of treatment can be summarized in the "Five R's": **R**elieving pain, **R**estoring function and ROM, **R**educing inflammation, **R**elaxing muscles, and **R**e-educating posture and movement. A good treatment plan will be multi-faceted to address each of these goals.

There are a number of treatment options available that can help you attain these goals. Pain relief can be accomplished through the use of medication, hydrotherapy, massage, and/or acupuncture; medication and hydrotherapy can also reduce inflammation. Massage therapists, occupational therapists, and physical therapists can work with you to restore ease and range of motion, relax your musculature, and help you develop healthier posture and less stressful ways of moving your body.

Most of the injuries that massage therapists sustain respond best to a combination of treatments. Since most of these injuries are syndromes that involve a number of different processes going on at once, each component needs to be addressed with a specific treatment. One treatment alone seldom completely resolves an injury. There are many treatments currently available that have been found to be effective in treating RSI's. Some of them will be prescribed or recommended by your physician; others will be carried out by a physical therapist, occupational therapist, or massage therapist. The treatment method that works best for you is often found through trial and error. You and your physician or therapist may try some treatments that turn out to be completely ineffective, and then find some others that work very well for you. You may find that a treatment that worked well at one stage of your recovery no longer works at a more advanced stage, or vice versa. Staying flexible and open to experimenting with different treatments will help you have a more successful recovery.

Rest

Rest is universally recommended as the primary treatment for RSI's. Rest involves a cessation or decrease in activities that are causing or exacerbating your symptoms, as well as partial or total immobilization of the injured body part. For your injury to get better, you will have to stop doing the thing that got you injured in the first place.

In almost all cases where injury is a result of doing massage, you will need at least to cut down on the amount of massage you do to allow the affected tissues to heal. If you are badly injured, your physician may recommend that you curtail all strenuous use of your hands, including massage, for a period of time. Your physician may also suggest that you keep the injured area still to encourage rest, and may prescribe a splint (for the hand/wrist) or a sling (for the elbow) to accomplish this (see "Splinting" below). The extent of your injury will determine how much you will need to rest your hands to resolve the injury.

Rest is a relative term, and many physicians disagree upon how much rest to prescribe. Many experts argue that rest is beneficial only up to a point. Beyond that point, they assert that it can actually be detrimental. Disuse can cause muscle and tendon tissue to atrophy. Atrophy happens very quickly, often within a few weeks. Disuse also reduces circulation, which impedes healing. As a result of atrophy and reduced blood flow, the tissues become weak and irritable, and even the smallest motion can cause pain. Most doctors feel it is best to try to find a "happy medium," a balance between absolute rest and moderate activity. The most effective treatments seem to combine some amount of rest, perhaps including the use of splints, with an exercise program that sustains muscle tone and promotes adequate circulation.

Splinting

Splints are often used to stabilize the position of the hand and wrist to allow for healing and to protect against reinjury. If your injury was caused by wrist flexion, a splint will hold the wrist in a neutral position so the injury is not continually aggravated. A splint can also provide extra support for the joint during activity, cutting down the risk of stressing the joint and reinjuring the tissues in or around it.

Splints are made of a hard material such as plastic on one side that is held to the forearm and hand by straps on the other. Unlike a cast, a splint can be removed for exercise and movement of the injured area. Complete immobilization (casting) is a good treatment method for broken bones, not for soft tissue injuries. The bone needs to be held absolutely still during healing so that the scar tissue can mature, harden and shrink without being disturbed. It can then "weld" the bone back together. In a soft tissue injury, you definitely do not want the muscle or tendon tissue to heal solidly together, otherwise you would be left with little range of motion at the joint. Scar tissue in soft tissue needs to be minimized and kept flexible so it will not restrict motion. Combining the use of a splint with gentle mobilization and exercise can keep scar tissue from hardening and shrinking while also allowing the injury to rest.

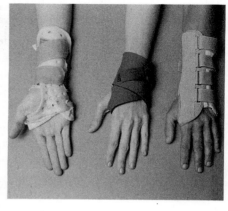

Photo 59

The use of splints for RSI's is yet another hotly debated topic. They are prescribed routinely by many physicians, physical therapists, and occupational therapists. Some conditions, like CTS, respond well to the use of wrist splints. CTS sufferers tend to wake up with sore hands and wrists in the morning from overflexing the wrists as they sleep, which puts pressure on the median nerve. Wearing splints at night can help keep the wrist straight, relieving pressure on the nerve. For other soft-tissue injuries, they can be a mixed blessing. While they are effective at allowing the injury to rest, over-dependency on or overuse of splints can cause atrophy and weakness, problems that can hinder your ability to heal.

There is a big difference between a "support" and a "splint." Supports are meant to offer extra stability to weak joints, not to rest injuries. Wrist and elbow supports and neoprene wraps can be bought over-the-counter at your pharmacy. They usually come in small, medium, and large sizes. If your wrist or elbow is somewhere between two sizes, the support may not fit well, and as a result can be ineffective. A poorly-fitting support can even aggravate your injury. A doctor, physical therapist, or occupational therapist can supply you with adjustable, better-quality splints and supports. Some insurance policies cover these appliances. Physical therapists and occupational therapists can create a splint for you which is custom fitted to your wrist or elbow. These tend to be the most effective and comfortable to wear. Unlike a support, a splint can keep the joint still, allowing it to rest and heal (Photo 59).

If you wear a splint for support and or rest, you will need to watch for diminished muscle size in the injured area. Make sure your physician, PT, or OT are aware of atrophy if you notice it is happening. If your injury is not severe, you should be able to take off the splint for some time each day and do exercises to keep the muscles toned. If you are severely injured, you may have to put up with some atrophy to get the benefit of resting the injured area. Your PT or OT will be able to prescribe some exercises or gentle mobilizations to do when she feels that you are ready for them.

Medications

Medication is often used to reduce inflammation and relieve pain from RSI's. There are two types of medicine that can achieve these effects. Which one you use depends on your injury and the recommendation of your doctor.

Non-steroidal anti-inflammatory drugs (NSAIDs)

Aspirin, ibuprofen and naproxyn (Aleve) are NSAIDs that are available over the counter. Acetaminophen, known by the brand name Tylenol, can relieve pain, but has no anti-inflammatory effect. Your doctor can prescribe prescription-strength NSAIDs that may be more effective than over-the-counter drugs. These include Ansaid, Nalfon, and Voltaren, among others. Each one of these is slightly different; it is sometimes necessary to try several before you find one that is effective for you. NSAIDs can be irritating or even damaging to the stomach, and some people cannot tolerate them. They are best taken with food to protect the stomach. Aspirin and other NSAID's do not interact well, and should not be taken at the same time.

These medications have to be used consistently to be effective in reducing inflammation. For example, taking ibuprofen sporadically for a few days will have little effect on your injury. Usually it takes a week or two for medication to start reducing the inflammation.

Anti-Inflammatory Steroids

Cortisone is a synthetic steroid used to reduce inflammation. Cortisone injections are a common treatment for tendinitis, and can be extremely effective. Often one injection in the right spot can clear up a mild or moderate tendinitis immediately. Cortisone injections for overuse syndrome, however, tend to have little to no effect. It is very important to have these injections done by a specialist, someone who is experienced in treating hands with cortisone and can get the medicine in exactly the right place. Cortisone does have significant side effects, and should therefore be used in moderation. With repeated use, cortisone can break down tendon tissue. One cortisone injection should have no systemic effect on your body. If your physician wants to do a series of injections, he will need to help you weigh the possible benefit to your injury against the possible harm that steroids can have on your tendons and the rest of your body.

Heat and Cold Therapy

Both heat and ice can be used effectively for treating RSI's. Generally, ice is used to treat acute injury where inflammation is present, and heat is used for chronic injury. The application of heat increases circulation to superficial tissues, which makes rigid, contracted muscle tissue more pliable and speeds healing. Ice causing temporary constriction of blood vessels, followed by an even greater increase in blood flow to the tissues than is produced by heat. Injuries in which inflammation plays a major role, like tendinitis/tenosynovitis, respond very well to ice treatments. When chronic muscle hypertonicity is a major factor, as in thoracic outlet syndrome, heat is often indicated and can be quite helpful in loosening up and relaxing muscle tissue. Heat can be applied to structures close to the skin using wet towels or pads (like Hydrocollator pads), and to deeper structures using ultrasound equipment. Ice therapy can involve direct ice massage, the use of ice packs, or ice water immersion.

Ice also can be used as a natural pain reliever. When you apply ice to the injured area, it becomes numb, and pain diminishes temporarily. There are several ways to apply ice, and ice packs are popular with PT's and OT's. However, some authorities recommend ice massage, or the direct application of ice to the skin over the affected area, instead of ice packs. Direct ice massage pinpoints specific areas of pain instead of freezing an entire area of tissue, which can cause reduced circulation to the area and impede healing.

Whether to apply heat or ice can be a tough call in many injuries. The musculature around the injury may be quite hypertonic; however, there may also be inflammation present. Some people respond better to ice than to heat, and vice versa. Listen closely to your body to see how you react to each kind of treatment. Your PT or OT will be able to determine which treatment is safe and advisable at a given time. If you would like to supplement the hydrotherapy treatments you receive from the PT or OT with home treatments, be sure to discuss this with them first (see Coping With Pain below) so you can coordinate your efforts with theirs and avoid overtreatment. When in doubt, ice is a safer bet than heat. Exercise care when using ice to avoid overfreezing your skin.

Contrast baths (vascular flush) can be very effective in treating chronic repetitive stress injuries. Alternately placing the affected area in moderately hot water and ice water maximizes blood flow to the injury site.

Massage Therapy

Muscle hypertonicity and spasm often accompany injury. The muscles surrounding an injury site contract and go into spasm in an attempt to "splint" and guard the injured area from further trauma. In overuse syndrome, constant muscular contraction is one of the features of the injury. Chronic muscle hypertonicity causes local ischemia and vasoconstriction, leading to more contraction, spasm and pain. Massage can be very effective treatment in relieving pain and increasing circulation to the injured area.

When the injury is acute, avoid massaging the injured area itself. Massage can irritate the area and cause more inflammation. Only massage therapists who have obtained extra training in injury treatment should work directly on the injured tissues. Instead, massage should be done to surrounding areas that may be contracted or in spasm. Gentle, passive mobilization of the injured area keeps the tissues flexible and helps prevent abnormal formation of scar tissue. Manual lymphatic drainage (MLD) techniques can also be done to facilitate removal of waste products from the damaged tissues. MLD is particularly effective in treating the chronic inflammation associated with RSI's. Once most of the inflammation is resolved, massage in the injured area can be effective in breaking up and realigning scar tissue to restore full range of motion.

The value of full-body, relaxation massage in healing should not be overlooked. A person who is injured and dealing with chronic pain can become very tense and irritable. The injury affects their entire being, not just their arm. The overall tension that builds up can exacerbate their symptoms. Getting a massage purely for relaxation and comfort can be tremendously therapeutic both in terms of healing and pain relief.

Physical therapists (and some occupational therapists and advanced massage therapists) do a type of deep tissue massage that uses deep, cross-fiber frictioning technique to break up adhesions and realign scar tissue, and also lengthen contracted muscles. Little to no lubrication is used, and deep work is initiated immediately without warming up the tissues. Although the treatment can be quite painful, it can be quite effective when applied in moderation.

Exercise, Stretching and Mobilization

Many experts feel that exercise should be started as early as possible in injury treatment. Some physical therapists feel that you should start exercising as soon as you can do mild exercise without pain. Exercise counteracts muscle atrophy from disuse, and stretching and mobilization help restore ROM and discourage abnormal scar tissue formation. Your physical or occupational therapist will design an exercise program tailored to your needs. Stick to this program, and do not supplement it with your own exercises. Some exercises or stretches may be counterproductive and contraindicated at certain points in your treatment.

Do not do strengthening exercises on your own when you are first injured. The repetitiveness of strengthening exercises may in itself can exacerbate your injury. It is often difficult to determine the right time to start exercise. Rely on your physical or occupational therapist to help you decide when the right time has arrived.

Stretches and passive mobilization are begun in the early stages of treatment. As your injury begins to heal and inflammation starts to subside, exercise will be added. When you first begin treatment, the PT, OT, or massage therapist will do these for you and you will be passive.

Neural tension is thought to be a contributing factor to overuse syndrome, carpal tunnel syndrome and thoracic outlet syndrome. Relieving some of this tension by stretching the three major nerves of the arm may be helpful in preventing these injuries. Check with your physician and/or physical therapist/occupational therapist to see if these stretches could be helpful in treating your injury.

As your treatment progresses, you will be assigned exercises and stretches to do at home. Your PT or OT will prescribe the exercises, but it's up to you to do them consistently. Most likely, part of the reason you were injured was that your muscles were too weak to withstand the intensity of the work that was demanded of them. Unless you strengthen those muscles, you will not be up to the demands of doing massage. A massage "athlete" understands the vital role that exercise plays in her life and in her career. Once you are out of physical or occupational therapy, it will be important to maintain and eventually increase your level of fitness and strength to keep from being reinjured.

Surgery

Surgery is usually a last resort. There is usually no need to rush into surgery, except in cases where nerve damage may occur if an injury is not resolved quickly. Some surgical techniques have been found to be quite effective in treating certain repetitive stress injuries. In the case of true carpal tunnel syndrome that has not responded to more conservative treatments, surgery can completely cure the nerve impingement. For other conditions, surgery is completely ineffective. Surgery is seldom indicated as a treatment for non-specific muscle/tendon injury classified simply as overuse syndrome, since it is ineffective and may cause more problems than it solves. In the hand, the intrusion of surgical instruments into the small spaces and delicate structures can cause damage that can have worse consequences than the original injury. This has to be weighed against the possible benefits of the surgery.

Before considering any surgery, make sure you have an exact diagnosis of your injury. Get a second opinion from another physician or surgeon who specializes in upper extremity repetitive stress injury. Expect to go through a period of rehabilitation after surgery to restore function, strength, and ROM to the affected limb.

Alternative Treatments

A growing number of people look to alternative health care to treat injury. The alternative therapies most commonly used for injury treatment and management are chiropractic, massage and bodywork, acupuncture and Chinese medicine, homeopathy, and naturopathy.

Many persons find the treatment they receive from alternative healthcare providers to be as, if not more, effective than traditional treatment methods. The benefits of massage therapy have been discussed in some detail above. The massage therapist who is experiencing symptoms of injury is best advised to see either an M.D., N.D., or D.O. before seeking alternative treatment. Discuss alternative therapy options with your doctor and make sure that she knows that you are seeking other types of care so she can coordinate her treatment accordingly. An increasing number of doctors are happy to have their patients try alternative treatments as an adjunct to medical treatment. The ultimate decision as to the type of treatment you wish to pursue is, of course, yours to make.

Coping With Your Injury During Treatment and Recovery

When you are injured, more than just your hand or arm need to be treated. This type of injury affects your whole life, and can be very difficult to deal with emotionally. You may be in pain some or all of the time, making you irritable, short-tempered and preoccupied. Your work may be interrupted, causing serious economic hardship. Your family may be less than completely supportive of your situation, which can leave you feeling abandoned. If your recovery takes a long time, you may lose hope at times. As a result of these situations, you may experience a number of conflicting emotions -- anger, sadness, frustration, despair -- that can lead to anxiety and depression. Depression is, in fact, a very common side effect of injury. Symptoms of depression include feelings of hopelessness, lethargy, inability to carry out daily activities, uncontrolled and/or constant crying, and loss of interest and enthusiasm for life. These symptoms should be carefully monitored. If they last more than one or two weeks, you should seek professional help. Left untreated, depression can interfere with your body's ability to heal and hinder the treatment of your physical symptoms. There are several steps you can take to keep your spirit in good shape as you move toward health during treatment.

See a Counselor

It is impossible to properly treat your body without also addressing your emotions. One of the most important things we learn as massage therapists is that the body and mind cannot be separated: what you do with one affects the other. A counselor can help you bring these two pieces of the puzzle together. A well-trained counselor can help you work out your feelings about your injury and how it is affecting your life. During a difficult or lengthy recovery period, it can be very reassuring to have someone in your life who is focused on your well-being and is always on your side. A good counselor can offer you encouragement, perspective, and compassion more consistently and objectively than even the best-meaning friend or family member. Occupation-related injury can be very upsetting; having someone to rely on as you deal with it is invaluable. A sympathetic counselor can help you retain a positive attitude that can speed your healing process.

A counselor can also help you deal with your feelings about how and why you were injured. Many massage therapists feel that they were injured because they failed in some way: if only they were better persons or better therapists, the injury would not have happened. Hopefully, the information in this book will help you realize that injury is an occupational hazard of doing massage that affects most massage therapists, not a sign of incompetence as a therapist and certainly not an indication that you are a bad person. This attitude can damage your self-esteem, or be an indication that your self-esteem was not very strong to begin with. A trained counselor can help you sort out these feelings, so that you can regain a healthy self-image.

If you are under a great deal of stress, your counselor may suggest some relaxation techniques such as meditation or guided imagery in addition to your sessions. She may also recommend that ask your doctor to prescribe a tranquilizer or muscle relaxant to help you cope better. Stress impedes healing, and should be reduced as much as possible while you are recuperating. If you have been feeling anxious and/or depressed consistently for more than a few weeks, you should consider asking your doctor about anti-depressant medication as well. Depression that is not treated can become a chronic problem. You are suffering enough just by being injured; do not hesitate to get the emotional help you need.

Form a Support Group

Another way of coping emotionally is to seek out other injured massage therapists and form a support group. You may feel alone with your injury, and it is reassuring to know that there are many other massage therapists who are going through the same experience. You can find other injured massage therapists by putting a notice in your massage school's newsletter or on their bulletin board. You can also contact your state or city chapter of the American Massage Therapy Association (AMTA) and enlist their help in your search. There are so many injured massage therapists, it should not be difficult to find others who will be willing to get together with you and share their experiences and feelings.

Coping with Pain

Pain relief is important on both a comfort level and on a healing level. If you have been in constant pain for a considerable amount of time, you may almost forget what it is like to not be in pain. Your muscles and nervous system are in a continuous state of vigilance, waiting to defend you when the next wave of pain hits. Relieving pain, even if it is only for a an hour or two, reminds your body what "normal" and "healthy" feel like. Once you remember that feeling, you can work more effectively toward health and normalcy.

As mentioned above, methods used to reduce inflammation, such as medication and ice therapy, are also very effective at relieving pain. Massage can relax stiff, tense, sore muscles and restore a feeling of well-being. Guided imagery, meditation and other relaxation techniques can help you deal with pain and stress. Many people swear by acupuncture for its pain-relief benefits.

Take Care of Yourself!

While you are undergoing treatment, you need to do everything you can to take good care of yourself in general. Many persons find that they feel extremely tired when they are injured. Fatigue is a natural reaction to pain and trauma, a way for your body to let you know that you need to slow down to facilitate healing. Make sure you get plenty of rest, eat well, and exercise lightly. Give yourself a break, and let yourself heal.

Stay in Charge of Your Treatment and Recovery

The ultimate power in the process of rehabilitation lies with you. Ask any questions that come up, even if they seem insignificant. Write them down before your appointments, if necessary, so you will be prepared. Ask what kind of results you can expect from treatment, and an estimate of how long the treatment might take. Usually it is not possible to predict exactly how much time an injury will take to heal, but you should be given some idea of when you might expect to start seeing improvement. You still need to monitor your own progress. If you feel you are not getting better or a particular treatment is not working, ask your physician, PT, or OT to reassess your treatment and discuss other options with you. Be your own advocate. If you are seeing a number of practitioners (PT, OT, doctor, LMP, etc.) all at once, you will need either to coordinate your care yourself or ask one of the practitioners (usually your primary care physician) to coordinate for you. Otherwise you may end up duplicating treatments, aggravating your condition. Taking an active, instead of passive, role in your recovery will make you feel empowered and aid in your recovery.

Keep Your Expectations Realistic

Most RSI's take time to develop, sometimes months or years. Accordingly, they usually take a long time to heal. Understandably, injured massage therapists want to heal as quickly as possible so they can go back to a normal life and practice. They often want a "quick fix," a fast solution that will get them back to work or school as soon as possible. Certain treatments, like cortisone injections, may relieve symptoms quickly, fooling you into thinking that you are cured and can resume using your hands or arms the way you used to. If you resume your activities before the injury has had a chance to heal completely, you will end up reinjuring yourself. Going back to square one when you thought you were better is even more frustrating and injurious than being conservative and waiting for true healing to occur. There are no quick and easy answers for these problems. Try to think of your recovery in terms of months rather than weeks. If you were injured badly enough, it may take years to get back to normal. You may even have lasting, permanent effects from the injury.

Until you are sure that you can handle normal activity without reinjuring yourself, play it safe. That may mean taking time off from school, or reducing your workload considerably for some time. If you rely on massage for your livelihood, you will be understandably reluctant to decrease your massage workload to accommodate healing time. You may feel that you cannot afford to do so. The question is: can you afford *not* to? Continuing to massage while you are injured, or resuming massage work before you are healed, can lead to more injury and serious, long-term disability. If you lose the use of your hands, you may not be able to do *any* kind of work. You must always weigh the short-term gain against the long-term consequences. It is better to take a short break now and save yourself future pain and loss of income.

Getting Back Into Massage After An Injury Has Healed

When you resume your massage work after any period of rest, make sure you gradually increase the number of massages you do. Start out doing very few massage with at least a few hours in between each massage. After a period of injury treatment, you will need to be even more conservative, especially if you were severely injured. Your PT, OT, or physician should be able to prescribe a preliminary work schedule that will allow you to slowly get used to doing massage again. To take the most conservative possible approach, start with a five-minute massage and see if you feel any pain or discomfort. If not, you can extend this massage by five minute increments as long as you remain acutely aware of any adverse reaction. If you start to feel pain or discomfort at any point, stop immediately. You will have found your limit at that time. Do not do any massage the next day to allow for healing, and reduce any inflammation that may have occurred from doing massage with ice or medication. Then repeat the experiment.

It may take quite a while to build back up to the number of massages you were doing before you were injured. Some massage therapists, particularly those who were severely injured, may find that they cannot do as many massages as they used to do before they begin to feel pain. If this is the case for you, you will need to adapt your work life to accommodate the aftereffects of your injury. Massage may become a part-time career, instead of full-time, which you supplement with other kinds of work (as long as the other work is not hand-intensive). If you are able eventually to resume your original massage schedule, do not let allow yourself to forget the lessons you learned when you were injured. Remember also that a history of injury makes you more likely to be injured again (see Chapter 2). Consider this a new beginning, an opportunity to learn from past mistakes, a chance to incorporate injury awareness and prevention into your massage work.

9

(re)Designing Your Life and Work to Prevent Injury

Many aspects of your life and work affect your ability to prevent injury. You use your upper extremity almost constantly every day. Even in your sleep, the position in which you hold your hands and arms can contribute to injury. To stay healthy, you must try to incorporate body awareness into all areas of your life and work. This task is actually easier than it sounds. Once you are more aware, you will find that this consciousness becomes an integral part of the way you live your life. You will begin to notice many potentially harmful activities that you used to do without thinking, and start adapting them to be easier on your hands.

Protect Your Hands Every Day

There is an old story about a famous violinist who was so protective of his hands that he never used them in his daily life. Other people fed him, opened doors for him, chauffeured him around: all to save his precious hands and fingers for the more important work of playing the violin. Of course, this violinist went to a rather neurotic extreme to save his hands. Most massage therapists have no choice but to use their hands and arms in their daily lives in addition to doing massage work. However, you can be careful about the way you use your hands to reduce or eliminate some everyday stresses that could increase your chance of injury. You can greatly reduce your risk of injury by reducing the amount of manual labor you do and by avoiding using your hands in an unnecessarily stressful manner.

In fact, the neurotic violinist was not completely wrong in his approach to injury prevention. It is reasonable to ask others in your life to do *some* things for you that might be overly stressful to your hands. If you have a partner or a housemate, you can certainly ask them to open stuck jar tops or frozen faucets for you. Remember that part of body awareness is acknowledging your weaknesses or limitations in addition to your strengths. You are only human. Admitting this fact and asking for help will keep you healthy.

A number of day-to-day activities commonly done with the hands can be done with other parts of the body. For example, most people open doors with their hands. Unless a door has a knob that must be turned, you can push it open with your shoulder or your foot. You may be able to find electric devices to do some work that you currently do with your hands. Stop using your bare hands to do tasks that could be done with a tool designed for that purpose. Turning, twisting, or wrenching things open with your hands may be macho, but it is also unnecessary and potentially harmful.

Massage therapists with upper extremity injuries often complain that their car becomes a torture chamber for them if they have manual steering, manual windows, or a manual transmission. If they can afford to, massage therapists would be well advised to buy cars with power steering, power windows, and automatic transmission so that driving does not become yet another taxing activity for the upper extremity.

Carrying heavy objects can be stressful to your arms and hands. A steel pot filled with cold water that is carried by a long handle can put a tremendous strain on the forearm of the person carrying it. Supporting some of the weight by placing the other hand underneath the pot at the same time will distribute the weight between the two arms. If the pot is hot, either use a potholder to support the bottom, or let it stay on the stove and empty the contents into a serving bowl or your plate. When carrying packages, distribute the weight between the two arms. If your package has long enough handles, carry it on your forearm or your shoulder to avoid gripping the handles with your hands. These may seem like very small points, but the cumulative effect of all of this extra manual activity can be substantial.

To maintain your overall physical condition, it is important to remain active. Participating in sports is a great way to get exercise. It can also be a great way to hurt your hands. Sports that use the upper extremity extensively, like tennis, are best avoided. Other sports that can easily traumatize the hands, like rock climbing, may not be a good idea either. Of course, it is your choice which sports you want to continue doing. If you wish to play tennis, make sure your arms are strong enough to withstand the impact of the ball and the repetitive motion of the racquet before you start playing. Protect your hands with gloves when you climb, and treat any trauma immediately and completely. Even seemingly innocuous sports like bicycling can traumatize the hands. Gel-padded handlebar grips and gloves can cushion the vibration and impact of uneven terrain on your hands and arms.

Other activities aside from sports can traumatize the hands. Repetitive activities that cause sharp impact to the hands, like hammering nails and stapling papers, should be avoided or reduced as much as possible. Your hands are your livelihood; you don't want to do anything that bangs them, hits them, pinches them, vibrates them, or traumatizes them in any way.

Chapter 2 discussed how massage overuses the hands. To avoid compounding this problem, try not to do other hand-intensive activities either as vocations or hobbies. A professional massage therapist who chooses to do computer work to supplement her income greatly increases her risk of repetitive stress injury. Much as we would like to feel that we can do anything we want in life, there are real limits to how much use and abuse our upper extremities can take. Playing an instrument semi-professionally or building furniture by hand as a hobby in addition to your massage work can push you over the edge from health into injury. Go easy on your hands and arms -- they are the only ones you will ever have!

Dealing with the Demands of School

While you are a student, you will need to be very careful about the way you work in order to stay healthy. Students are prone to injury because they have not yet had the time or experience to develop good body mechanics. When you do massage as a student, limit yourself to working only under the most ideal situations. You have this luxury while you are in school -- take advantage of it! Make sure your physical work environment is set up for your comfort and ease. Review the potentially harmful work situations in Chapter 2 and avoid them as much as possible.

Most massage students are required to do only a few massages each week while they are in school. Volunteer opportunities and externships/internships may be made available to you as a student that will require you suddenly to increase the number of massages you do and decrease the amount of time you leave between massages. In this new, more professional situation, you will likely feel pressured to do more work than you are comfortable doing. The pressure will also overide your self-awareness. Enter into these situations with great caution. They can be wonderful introductions to the world of professional massage, but they can also be a fast road to injury.

Similarly, be prudent about taking hands-on workshops to learn new or different techniques and approaches to massage in addition to your school work. Workshops are usually designed to cover a large body of information in a short amount of time. As a result, they can be physically demanding. You may be required to do many hours of hands-on massage during the workshop. New techniques you learn may feel awkward, or may throw off your normal body mechanics. This sudden increase in the amount of massage you are doing, combined with the introduction of new techniques, will increase your chances of being injured. Limit yourself to one workshop per month. Try to take workshops during your school break, or when you expect to have an easy week. Stay alert to any signals your body may send you during the workshop that you are overdoing it. If you get tired, or start feeling any pain or discomfort, tell the instructor you need to sit out and observe for a while.

Students often feel pressured to keep up in school and show that they can do any technique they are taught. This pressure can make you afraid to tell your instructors that you are having symptoms of injury, uncomfortable in a particular work environment or awkward when doing certain techniques. Peer pressure can also make you reluctant to say you hurt, for fear of what your fellow students will think of you.

It is very important that you speak up for yourself and let your instructors know that you need help. The instructor cannot help you unless he knows that something is wrong. He will most likely be very sympathetic and help you find alternative ways of massaging that will be more comfortable for you. If you tell him you are injured, he may be able to offer some good advice, including a referral to a health care practitioner who can help you decide on a treatment plan. You can also ask him to keep your injury confidential, so you will not have to deal with the potentially insensitive comments of others. In the unlikely event that your instructor is not receptive to your needs, you can always ask another instructor or a school administrator to intervene and address you problem.

Remember that the ultimate responsibility for your health rests with you. You must be your own advocate. Have the courage to do whatever it takes to keep your hands and arms healthy. Take time off from school if you need to. Interrupting your schooling may be upsetting and frustrating, but it is better than developing an injury that can shorten, limit, or end your massage career. Injuries that start in school tend to continue and worsen with the demands of professional employment. Protect your training, your new career, and your quality of life by dealing with injury swiftly, responsibly, and completely.

Making Awareness Part of Your Work Routine

Before you do your first massage of the day, you probably do some things to get ready for the work ahead. You check to see how many massages you do that day. You make sure that you have enough sheets and oil for your clients, and that the room and table are set up properly. Whether you are a student or a professional, simply add body awareness into your pre-massage preparations to start preventing injury before you even touch a client.

Take a few minutes to assess your physical and emotional readiness to do massage. Ask yourself: how do I feel today? Do my hands or arms hurt or ache, do they feel tight, or weak, or do they feel good today? How do I feel in general: tired or rested, full of energy or sluggish, warm or cold, peaceful or anxious, happy or down? Note any factor that could increase your risk for injury that day, and make a quick plan of how you will deal with those factors during the day so they don't put you at risk for injury. If you are tired or sluggish, perhaps you can find a time between clients to take a short nap to recharge. Think about keeping a spray bottle filled with water and lemon slices next to the table, and spraying a fine mist over your face to refresh yourself as you work. If you are seriously tired and not feeling up to seeing so many clients that day, perhaps you can consider rescheduling one or two for a different day. If you are anxious and/or unhappy, try to do something that will relax you and put you at ease. Perhaps listening to a certain kind of music, or taking a warm foot bath with lavender oil in the water will make you feel better. Maybe meditating before you start your workday would make you more peaceful. Doing some vigorous exercise for fifteen minutes to half an hour could be very calming, and will also get your circulation going if you feel cold.

To be ready physically for your first massage, you will need to warm up your body, your hands, and your arms. Many massage therapists notice that their hands are cold when they first begin a massage. Cold hands are an indication that circulation is not flowing sufficiently through the arms and hands. As you read earlier, lack of circulation will make your muscles rigid and more likely to tear and impede your ability to heal. Always warm up before you do your first massage of the day, after any lengthy break, or whenever your hands are cold.

Start your day with some of the muscle stretches in Chapter 7. Remember that your muscles may be cold and sluggish, so stretch gently. Follow your stretches with a five minutes of light aerobic exercise, like running in place, jumping rope or dancing.

Just as you would swim a few easy laps before swimming a race, or hit some balls lightly over the net before you played a tennis game, think of the first few minutes of each massage as part of your warm-up. Keep your techniques easy and light (little pressure): perhaps some broad, light effleurage strokes with the hands, some with the forearms to warm up your hands and arms at the same time as you warm up your client's tissues. Only begin to do deeper, more stressful techniques when your hands are warm and you are feeling energized.

Make time to relax, stretch and breathe consciously throughout the day. No matter how good your technique is, how good your body mechanics are, or how careful you are as you massage, periods of physical and mental work need to be balanced with periods of rest, relaxation and exercise if you are to stay healthy. It is also important to maintain a healthy lifestyle, eat a healthy diet, and get enough sleep. Doing 30 massages per week, with a five-day work week without getting enough sleep, rest, and exercise during that week is likely to get you injured.

Counteract the stress and physical tension of your work by receiving massage. As you know, massage is very effective as a preventive measure to reduce your risk of injury. Find a colleague who will exchange massages with you and see her regularly, at least once per week. You can also massage your own forearms and hands at the end of each work day. Use your forearms to create the strokes, since you need to rest your overused hands. Here is a simple self-massage routine you can use: lay your forearm and hand on a desk in front of you with the palm facing up. Apply a good amount of oil or lotion to your forearm. Place your left forearm at the medial epicondyle of the elbow, and make a long, even stroke down the flexor muscles to the wrist (Photo 60). Flex your wrist, and grab the folds of skin and fascia now apparent at the wrist with your left forearm. As you stroke back up the forearm flexors, let the hand slowly lower back down to the desk as you progress back to the medial elbow. Do these strokes several times, starting with light pressure and gradually increasing to moderate pressure. Turn the right forearm over so the palm is now facing the desk. Place your left forearm at the lateral epicondyle of the elbow and stroke down the extensor muscles to the wrist (Photo 61). Extend your wrist, and grab the folds of skin and fascia with your left forearm. As you stroke back up the forearm extensors, let the hand slowly lower back down to the desk as you progress back to the medial elbow. Again, do these strokes several times, increasing the

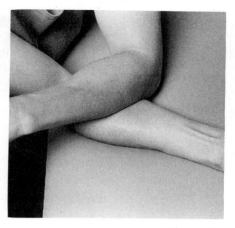

Photo 60

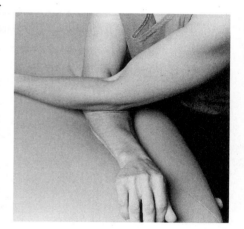

Photo 61

pressure as you go. Next, do some circular Lomi Lomi strokes on both sides of the arm (see Chapter 6). You can use your elbow for direct pressure to the muscles, but be very careful to avoid nerves and blood vessels, particularly in and around the forearm flexor muscles. Repeat this routine on the other arm. Remember that self-massage should not take the place of getting a professional, full-body massage; rather, it should be done as an additional, daily way to relax the arms.

Try to maintain this level of injury prevention awareness throughout the day. Be consistent, and this way of working will quickly become automatic. Expect that you may have to compensate for changes and surprises as the day unfolds. You will probably feel different at 3:00pm than at 9:00am. Each client will have his own particular effect on your mood, and therefore on your ability to protect yourself from injury. Some clients may be very demanding, while others may be very passive. Adjust the way you work for each client, just as you adjust your table height to accommodate the width of each client's body and the different techniques you want to use. Flexibility is a healthy quality that allows you to accommodate new and changing circumstances in your work.

Managing Your Professional Life to Avoid Injury

Chapter 2 discusses the importance of keeping a fairly consistent workload, since sudden increases in the number of massage you do is one of the leading causes of occupation-related injury in massage therapists. In actual practice, the number of massage you do each week is likely to vary, particularly while you are first setting up your practice. If you are a professional massage therapist and work in a clinic or salon situation, your workload may be controlled by your employer and the facility's receptionist. How then do you protect yourself from injury?

If you are self-employed, you are in control of how many massages you do and how much time you leave between massages. You can make sure you gradually increase the number of massages you do until you reach a work level that is comfortable and sufficiently profitable. When scheduling your clients, try to space them out to maintain a consistent workload. Do not let economic factors rule your decisions about workload. You may make more money in the short run, but you may also endanger your long-term ability to practice massage in doing so. Decide in advance what your work limit will be for any particular week, and stick to it. Keep a list of other massage therapists to whom you can refer potential clients if you cannot see them because your schedule is too full that day or week, especially if you are tired or your arms are feeling overused. If the client has a pressing need for a massage, she will appreciate the referral. Tell her you hope she will call you again in the future and you will likely keep her business.

It is admittedly more difficult to regulate your workload if you work for someone else. Many employers are not well-informed about massage-related injury, and may therefore have unreasonable expectations of their employees. It will be up to you to set very clear limits. Make your employer aware of your current workload limits when you first start working for her. If you are just starting out in massage, your limit may be fairly low. Tell your employer that you would like to start out with a small number of massages and slowly, gradually increase that number as you are able to. Impress upon her that you would like to work toward developing a schedule that will be profitable for her and healthy for you, and you need her help to do that. After all, she is counting on your productivity to make her money. If you become injured, you will not be any good to her.

Educate your employer about the prevalence of occupation-related injury among massage therapists and the need to create working conditions that help keep employees healthy. Show him this book, if you feel that would be helpful. Capture his attention by telling him that he can reduce expensive employee turnover by implementing some simple, inexpensive injury prevention methods into his business. Make him aware that worker's compensation insurance claims for injuries sustained on the job can cost employers a great deal of money. Get your fellow employees together and suggest a meeting with the employer to discuss optimizing working conditions. If your employer does not have the time or inclination to meet with you, write up a group proposal for the changes and limitations you wish to suggest. As a general guideline, you should have a minimum of fifteen minutes between one-hour massages, ten minutes between half hour massages (*in addition* to the time needed for the client to dress and for you to change the sheets). Set individual limits for number of massages per day and per week. If there is more work than the present number of massage therapists on staff can handle safely, suggest hiring more therapists. Ask your employer to develop a list of massage therapists in the community who can be called upon to substitute for staff who need to take time off to rest an injury. Make suggestions for improving the physical conditions of your workplace: rooms big enough to move comfortably around the table, or installation of hydraulic or electric tables. Be positive, enthusiastic, and firm and your employer may actually listen to you and adopt your suggestions.

Whether you work for yourself or for someone else, limit the length of your massages to one hour. An increasing number of individual massage therapists and clinics are offering longer massages, anywhere from one and one half hours to three hours. Luckily, the industry standard is still one hour. A one-hour massage is stressful enough; the more time you add without a break, the higher your risk of injury will be. You also may overtreat your client, leaving them feeling weak and drained instead of energized and well. Trying to resolve every complaint in one massage usually does not work. It took a while for your client to develop all that hypertonicity and pain; it is likely to take a number of treatments, plus re-education of the client, to help these symptoms go away. It is healthier and more realistic for you and your client to develop a *treatment plan* together that spaces out a number of massages over a two to six weeks. At the end of that time you can re-evaluate the client's condition (and perhaps check in with the other health care practitioners she is seeing) to assess the need for further treatment.

Most working massage practitioners seek additional training in techniques and approaches to massage during their professional life. Membership in a professional association, or state licensing statutes may require you to take a certain number of hours of continuing education each year. Professionals must be careful about taking hands-on workshops in addition to their usual workload, since this extra use of your hands is likely to overstress your upper extremity. Limit yourself to no more than one hands-on workshop per month, decrease the number of professional massages you do around the time of the workshop, and be on the lookout for any symptoms that may develop while you are participating in the workshop.

Develop a Realistic Attitude Toward Massage

The title "therapist" can be burdensome to those who do massage. They may have an image in their minds of someone who is perfect, never makes any mistakes, and can fix all problems. The pressure of living up to this image can make a massage therapist very self-conscious, self-doubting, and self-critical. When you bring the stress and tension of this attitude to your massage work, you lose the objectivity and clarity of mind necessary to be self-aware and protective of your health.

Try to develop a realistic, easy-going approach to massage. Therapists, whether massage, psychological, physical or occupational, are only human beings. There are limits to what you can do for your clients, no matter how "perfect" you try to be. You cannot "cure" your clients all by yourself -- they have to help in the process. It really is enough to do what you can for people, and let them take the rest of the responsibility. Accepting the limitations of what you can do for others is another part of the awareness that will keep you from being injured.

Dropping unreasonable expectations of yourself will allow you to relax and regain some perspective on your work. You will be better able to accept the information and suggestions in this book and let them become part of the way you live and work. You will become more flexible, more willing to try different ways of working that may be more comfortable for you and ultimately save you from being injured. You will develop your own, individual style that emphasizes your strengths and compensates for your limitations.

Remind yourself to lighten up as you work. Don't exhaust yourself in every massage. Think beyond what you want to achieve at the moment so you do not lose track of what you want to achieve in the session as a whole. Then pace yourself so you do not use up all your energy in the first ten minutes. A great massage does not have to include every technique you were ever taught. It also does not have to mean using a lot of force or pressure. Many times, a lighter touch can be just as effective, sometimes even more effective in treating certain complaints for certain people. Remember that treatment has to do with your *focus*, not the particular technique or amount of pressure you use. Educate your clients to understand that there are many therapeutic massage techniques that do not use much pressure. Help them open their minds and bodies to different ways of working that may turn out to be quite beneficial to their health and well-being.

Learn to set limits with your clients. Many massage therapists find it difficult to say "no" to their clients, even if saying "yes" means hurting themselves. These therapists are afraid that if they refuse to do a certain technique that causes them pain or that they feel is unsafe for their hands, the client will never come back to see them. This inability to set limits with clients often leads to injury.

Having a strong sense of personal boundaries and limits is healthy in any relationship. It is also an important element of professionalism. It is contrary to the therapeutic process to hurt yourself in order to help someone else. This kind of masochism sets up a martyr dynamic between you and your client that will make both you and him uncomfortable and tense. You must realize that your clients do not come to you because you do that one stroke with your thumb that they love. Most use a number of criteria to choose a massage therapist, the techniques he uses being just one of those criteria. You are more than the sum total of all your techniques. Your clients come to you because you are YOU, because they are comfortable with you, because they trust you. Being clear, firm and consistent about your personal and professional limits will help deepen that trust. A client who does not respond to that level of honesty and integrity probably would be better off with a different therapist.

Remember You Are Not Alone!

Injury prevention is a concern you share with all massage therapists. Enlist the aid and support of your colleagues to deal with this important issue. The camaraderie will help you maintain perspective and a sense of humor about this difficult subject. Your colleagues' encouragement will help you stay disciplined and consistent about staying in shape and taking care of yourself. Both students and professionals can benefit from group interaction about injury.

Meet with each other regularly for discussion and hands-on practice sessions. Talk about your injury concerns, whether they are symptoms you have developed, situations with clients that made you feel pressured or tense, or a new employer who wants you to increase your workload from 15 to 25 massages per week. Support each other's attempts to stand up for yourselves and protect your hands and arms. Encourage each other to take life and work less seriously, and make health and career longevity major priorities. In your hands-on practice session, watch each other work and point out potentially harmful habits. Offer constructive criticism about technique, and share new, less-stressful techniques you pick up in your work or from continuing education courses. Use this book as a guide for both discussion and hands-on work.

Many people find that it is difficult to keep to an exercise schedule. Forming an exercise class with your fellow therapists or fellow students can help motivate you to stick with your exercise routine. A group workout is much more fun than exercising alone. Get your group together three times each week and do the exercises and stretches in this book. Play music while you work out to help set a rhythm and keep you going. Take turns leading the class through the routine.

Redesigning your life and work to prevent injury is really about learning to be good to yourself. Taking responsibility for your own health and well-being is part of enhancing your self-respect and self-esteem. The best massage therapists are those who practice what they preach, who exude the kind of calmness and healthfulness that they are trying to instill in their clients. It is difficult to convince your clients to make health and well-being a priority when it is not a priority for you. Adapting our work and personal lives to allow room for health, relaxation, and peace of mind are challenges that all human beings face as modern life becomes increasingly complex and demanding. If we allow the well-being that massage promotes to permeate our own lives, we may be better able to handle all that the future holds in store.

In Conclusion

Massage is a challenging, demanding, and rewarding profession. It is certainly possible to have a long, successful career as a massage therapist if you give your own physical and emotional needs the same care and consideration that you do your clients'. Allow yourself to be human, to have strengths and weaknesses, to make mistakes, and to learn and grow from those mistakes. When you develop compassion for yourself, your compassion for your clients will deepen as well. The point where technique and compassion meet is where healing begins. Human beings have physical limits, and get injured if they push themselves too far past those limits for too long. Have enough respect for yourself to seek appropriate professional help when you are hurting, either physically or emotionally. Listen to your body, and become aware of the messages it sends you from moment to moment. This sensitivity will make your massages more subtle, artful, and effective. Become flexible in your thoughts and techniques, and you will be able to modify them quickly and easily in response to signals from your body and your client's body.

In my workshops, I have often felt that what massage students and therapists want more than anything from me is permission to relax and take care of themselves. I would like to offer all massage therapists permission to massage without pain. The most meaningful permission, however, is that which you give yourself. A massage career filled with joy instead of suffering is within your reach -- it is all up to you.

Appendix I
Will I Be Injured From
Doing Massage?

A short, unscientific quiz to increase your injury self-awareness.

Choose the answer that best describes you.

General Health Questions

1. I exercise:
   a. regularly (i.e., several times each week)
   b. sometimes or sporadically
   c. hardly ever or never

2. My age is:
   a. 18-29 years old
   b. 30-45 years old
   c. 46-60 years old

3. I have had pain/injury in my upper extremity, shoulders, neck or back in the past;
   a. never
   b. sometimes
   c. often

4. My general health is:
   a. great
   b. not bad
   c. poor

5. The joints in my hands/wrists are:
   a. very stable
   b. a little unstable (normal ROM)
   c. hypermobile

6. My posture is:
   a. great
   b. not bad
   c. poor

Questions about your life in general

7. I do other hand-intensive activities in addition to massage:
   a. hardly ever
   b. sometimes (e.g., occasional gardening, mountain bike riding, etc.)
   c. on a daily basis (e.g., I do computer work or play an instrument regularly)

8. I am careful about how I use my hands day-to-day:
   a. yes, very
   b. somewhat
   c. not really

9. I would assess my overall emotional state as:
   a. mostly calm and content
   b. under some stress
   c. *really* stressed out

Questions about your massage work:

10. When I massage, my body feels:
    a. comfortable, relaxed
    b. all right, but could be more relaxed
    c. uncomfortable, tense

11. When I massage, I am aware of keeping my wrists straight:
    a.   always
    b.   sometimes
    c.   never

12. I vary my strokes and the positioning of my client:
    a.   often
    b.   sometimes
    c.   not much

13. I use a great deal of pressure:
    a.   hardly ever
    b.   some of the time
    c.   most/all of the time

14. The part of the arm I use most in doing massage is:
    a.   my forearm/elbow
    b.   my full hand or fist
    c.   the tips of my fingers

15. I use my thumb:
    a.   hardly ever
    b.   some of the time
    c.   a good deal of the time

16. I breathe consciously while I massage:
    a.   often
    b.   sometimes (when I remember)
    c.   only to keep from passing out

17. The number of massages I do per week is:
    a.   1 - 5
    b.   6 - 15
    c.   I lost count around 20

18. The amount of time I leave between massages is:
    a. at least an hour
    b. ten minutes to half an hour
    c. just enough to change the sheets

19. If I feel pain in my hands during or after massaging, I:
    a. decrease my massage workload and see a doctor if it persists
    b. use ice/medication and watch to see if it persists, but do not decrease my workload
    c. ignore it until it gets bad

20. I rely on massage for:
    a. none of my living
    b. a portion of my living
    c. my entire living

SCORING:

each answer (a) = 3 points
each answer (b) = 2 points
each answer (c) = 1 point

Add up the points to find your final score.

Analysis of score:

50-60 points: Can't guarantee you will never be injured, but you are taking pretty good care of yourself. Keep it up!

40-49 points: You are taking more risks than you have to. Remember, you want a long, healthy career! Perhaps it is time to rethink lifestyle or massage habits?

39 or less: It is *definitely* time to make some changes so you can avoid becoming injured. It is never too late to start protecting yourself - **GO TO IT!**

Appendix II
Recommendations for
Massage Schools and Faculty

This is a challenging time to be teaching massage. The profession is growing very rapidly, and there is increasing pressure upon schools to produce professional massage therapists who are skilled and ready to meet the ever-greater demands of the workplace. It is no longer enough to teach Swedish relaxation massage, hygiene, and professional ethics in school. To stay competitive, schools must now include curricula on everything from trigger point therapy and shiatsu, to deep tissue and sports massage, to hydrotherapy and range of motion testing. They must also work many hours of anatomy, physiology, and clinical treatment into the students' already hectic schedule. This extensive material must be crammed into massage programs that are usually only six to eighteen months in length. Many school administrators and instructors feel they have barely enough time to cover this information, let alone to get into any of the subtleties or artistry of massage. And what about injury prevention? When students complain of pain, instructors can feel that there just is not enough time to find out what is causing the problem. Without guidance from instructors, these students can end up seriously injured. Without adequate information on self-care, *all* students remain at risk of serious injury, during their remaining time at school and later as professionals.

Schools and faculty are in a difficult situation. They want to provide the best training in the short amount of time available. They also care about their students, and want to help them adjust physically and emotionally to the demands of doing massage. How can we train good massage therapists who can compete in today's demanding massage market and arm them with the knowledge to stay healthy at the same time?

The answer for schools and faculty is much like the answer for individual massage therapists: we need to find a way to balance client care with self-care. The very nature of our profession is to promote health, to encourage others to take time out for self-awareness, self-care and rest. We need to send the same message to our students.

We also must make injury prevention a priority. Educators must rethink their curricula and make time to teach students what they need to know to stay healthy. Part of teaching a career is teaching people how to *live* that career. In a profession where most of the practitioners experience some kind of pain syndrome at some point in their careers, dealing with the possibility of injury during a professional training program is essential.

Students look to us for guidance about much more than just how to do massage techniques. They are too embroiled in their studies and too unaware of what awaits them in the professional arena to have any real perspective. They need us to help them gain objectivity and a sense of proportion about their work. Just as we teach students to have respect for their clients' boundaries and safety, we must teach them to have respect for their own boundaries and safety. As we teach them to understand and treat injury in their clients, we must teach them to do the same for themselves. Taking care of oneself is a learned behavior that can be taught in massage school. Massage educators can be important mentors who help their students grow both professionally and personally.

Recommendations

Schools and faculty can help their students prevent injury in several ways:

Speak Openly About Injury

Students need to hear directly from experienced massage therapists that injury is an occupational hazard of doing massage. They need to understand that massage is a physically demanding career. Instructors need to tell their students that many massage therapists experience symptoms of injury or impending injury during their careers. Bringing this issue out into the daylight will counteract the feelings of shame and inadequacy that keep students from telling their instructors about their symptoms, and from seeking proper care.

Teach Technique in Context

In our well-meaning attempt to teach students as many techniques as possible, we can end up producing massage therapists who have a large repertoire of techniques and little judgment about how to use them properly and safely. These therapists overtreat their clients and overuse their own upper extremities, which makes them prone to injury. Emphasizing humanity and artistry along with technique will help your students become mature, well-rounded professionals.

Schools and faculty can counteract this reliance on technique in several ways. First, we must teach technique in context from the very beginning of the training program. Many massage schools teach "routines," a series of specific techniques for each part of the body. Since these routines are not taught in the context of a particular client's complaints, students get the message that this is THE way to work on that part of the body. By the time the school curriculum starts asking students to match techniques to their client's real needs, the routines may already be ingrained. If the student is limited to an hour session in a professional setting, they may spend so much time doing all their routines that they never get to the parts that are bothering the client. It may seem obvious to the seasoned professional that routines are meant to be suggestions, not law. However, when we test students on these routines and reward them with a good grade if they do routines by rote, we reinforce them in the students' minds as simple, arbitrary solutions to every question.

To give a more contextual view of technique, the instructor can mention a common client complaint and then show various techniques (not a routine) that can be used to address the complaint. Encourage the student to be flexible and adaptive in his approach by asking for some other techniques that would work equally well for these complaints. Techniques that address the affected area in terms of the whole body can be taught alongside more area-specific techniques. Have the student say out loud what complaint she is addressing with each technique. This teaching method encourages critical thinking, and immediately connects techniques with helping the client, counteracting the tendency of the student to perform the same techniques indiscriminately on every client.

Teach Treatment as Intent, Not Technique

Chapter 1 discusses the confusion many students and professionals have as to what constitutes a "relaxation" technique and what constitutes a "treatment" technique. This confusion often arises in school. Some school curricula teach "Swedish relaxation" techniques for quite a while before introducing their students to "clinical treatment." Treatment is taught later in the program because the students do not learn about injury physiology until they have spent months on other more basic aspects of anatomy and physiology. Often the techniques used in the clinical curriculum are new, or different from those the student learned earlier in the program. They also tend to be repetitive, specific, and pressure-intensive, qualities that make them potentially harmful to the students' upper extremities. This way of teaching draws a distinction between techniques that are meant to relax the client and those that are meant to be therapeutic to the client. In the student's mind, relaxation techniques are broader, lighter strokes that cover large areas and tie in the whole body; treatment techniques are small, hand-intensive, repetitive movements that are applied to small areas.

Design your curriculum to present the concepts of relaxation and treatment as one and the same. It must be impressed upon the student that *any* technique can be therapeutic if it is the student's intent that it be so. If we can clarify this concept in the minds of our students, it will help counteract the tendency of massage therapists to feel they must use techniques that are stressful to their own bodies to have a therapeutic effect on their clients.

Teach Students to Vary Their Technique

Students also tend to get stuck in doing a particular technique with a particular part of their own bodies. For example, if they were taught to use their palms to friction down the erector spinae group, they will *always* use their palms for this part of the back. Varying the parts of the arm used in doing massage helps decrease the chances of injury. Try this exercise: have everyone start doing massages as they usually do. When you say "stop," everyone must do the technique they were just doing, but using a different part of their arm to do it. For example, say "stop," and tell everyone they must now use their elbow to do their last technique. If a student feels it is not appropriate to use the elbow in the particular area they were just massaging, ask him to explain why. Repeat this exercise a number of times during the session. It will help your students develop flexibility so they do not get into the habit of always using the same part of the arm or hand to do massage.

Encourage Students to Be Flexible

Make sure your students understand that coming up with another technique to use is not always the solution to every problem. Encourage your students to tell you "I don't know what to do next" while you are watching them do a massage, instead of rushing into another technique out of panic. Then you can discuss together the different options available to them. Reassure them that it is fine to do some broad effleurage strokes while they are thinking, strokes which are easy on their own body, feel nice to the client, and aid in lymphatic drainage. Help them focus on what the *client* needs in moments of indecision more than on their own fear of seeming hesitant. Let them know that they do not always have to be "doing" something during a massage, that they might need to simply rest for a moment and take a deep breath when they are feeling unsure how to proceed. Looking for options instead of seizing on technique introduces students to the subtleties of massage and encourages creativity and flexibility, elements that will help them stay healthy and enhance their skill as professionals.

Help Students Develop Healthy Attitudes About Massage

Chapters 2 and 9 discuss some of the common unrealistic expectations that massage therapists have of themselves and their work. These attitudes are sometimes picked up in massage school. Just as medical schools are getting away from handing down the "doctor as god" image from one generation of physicians to another, massage schools need to balance the "massage therapist as all-knowing healer" attitude with some reality checking. Help your students understand that they are only human, that they probably cannot "cure" all of their clients' ills, and that the client must participate in his own healing. Most importantly, make sure they get a very strong message about setting limits and maintaining boundaries with clients. Too many massage therapists feel that hurting themselves is an unavoidable part of helping their clients. We need to counteract this idea from the very first days of massage training if we are going to produce massage therapists who can handle themselves in a professional manner.

Continue to Stress a Whole-Body Approach to Massage

Educators and school administrators need to decide how they want to shape the massage profession. There is concern in some circles that the growing emphasis on area-specific treatment instead of whole-body treatment in our profession will soon make massage indistinguishable from physical therapy. It is important that we maintain the integrity of massage as a separate, legitimate approach to health. Instead of giving in to societal pressure to pigeonhole massage and make it more easily quantifiable, we need to educate the public that massage in its many forms has much to offer, both physically and spiritually, in ways that are different than other modalities. We need to teach our students the same thing, since they will be representing the massage profession to the public in the future.

Make whole-body involvement part of the way you teach massage. Teach students to balance time spent on individual techniques with time spent incorporating those techniques into a full-body massage. In testing situations, test for the ability to incorporate techniques holistically, not just for the ability to demonstrate techniques by themselves. What has made massage unique and popular for thousands of years is its ability to treat specific complaints and address the whole body at the same time. Eventually, we will have to find a happy balance between the specific and the holistic, since the emphasis on spot work is proving to be too stressful for many therapists.

Teach Treatment Planning, Not Just Treatment

Chapter 9 discusses the importance of teaching students to create a treatment plan to counteract the tendency to try to do too much in one massage. Instructors should impress upon their students that they cannot, and should not, try to resolve every complaint in one session. This point should be made not only to maintain the student's health, but also to counteract the public's idea that massage can be a quick fix. Massage therapists can offer the public a tremendous service by helping them become more realistic about what it takes to stay healthy. If our clients understand that maintaining health takes self-awareness and effort on their parts, they will have more realistic demands of massage therapists, relieving some of the pressure that causes us to become injured.

Train Teachers About Injury Prevention

Make sure your teachers are well-informed about massage-related injury. Train teachers to be on the lookout for warning signs of injury or impending injury in their students. Teachers are often unsure what and how much to say to students about injury. School administrators can help solve this dilemma by giving instructors a simple protocol to use in these cases. It can be as simple as telling instructors to take all complaints seriously, and recommend that students who are experiencing symptoms see their physician. Giving this kind of advice takes only a minute, and can make the difference between a student remaining healthy or suffering a debilitating, even permanent disability. Most importantly, let your students know on the first day of class that you are accessible and willing to talk to them if they start having any problems with their hands, arms, or any other part of their bodies.

Introduce Injury Prevention Information Early In Your Program

Massage students are generally quite ignorant about injury. They usually do not understand their own symptoms, have no idea when and if they should seek medical care, and know nothing about the potential for permanent damage if they continue to overuse their hands. Students can get injured at the very beginning of their training. The author has seen a number of first term students who are already complaining of pain and discomfort in their upper extremities. Equip your students with the facts they need early in your program so they can start protecting themselves from injury as soon as possible. As we all know, it is far easier to prevent injury in the first place than to treat it once it occurs.

Be Careful Not to Overload Your Students

Design your curriculum to allow students to gradually increase the amount of hands-on massage work they do. As discussed in Chapter 2, a sudden increase in massage workload can precipitate an injury. Be judicious in suggesting volunteer opportunities, workshops and internships/externships. Before accepting a student into an internship or externship program, find out if the student has experienced any pain or discomfort while she has been in school. Realize that she may be hesitant to admit any problem to you for fear that you will think she is not a "good" student. You may want to check in with her teacher and see if he has noticed any symptoms of injury. Explain to the student that taking on the extra work of an internship/externship can aggravate any symptoms she may already be experiencing and cause injury.

There is, of course, a limit to how much you can protect your students from injury. It is ultimately *their* responsibility to look after their own health. In years to come, however, it will be important for schools to be able to document their efforts to ensure the safety of their students. Corporations have recently been implicated in litigation brought against them by their employees for repetitive stress injury. It will not be long before schools offering professional training programs will be the target of similar litigation.

School administrators and instructors do so much already to help students successfully get through school. The logical next step is to make injury prevention and awareness part of these efforts. All the classes and training we can offer will have been meaningless if students are too injured to practice massage when they graduate. I encourage school administrators and faculty to work together to incorporate comprehensive information on injury awareness/prevention into their school's curriculum. I am available to help schools in this process, and to train instructors to identify and deal with injury in their students. It is quite simple, and inexpensive, to institute methods to safeguard your students. You may contact me through Infinity Press (see back cover) for more information.

Appendix III
Glossary of Terms

adhesions:	patches of scar tissue that have glued soft tissue structures to each other
anterior:	pertaining to the front of the body
congenital:	present at birth
contraindication:	a symptom or condition that precludes normally recommended treatment
dorsal:	pertaining to the back of the forearm
edema:	abnormal fluid accumulation in soft tissues
etiology:	cause of a disease or illness
hypermobile:	possessing excessive range of motion
hypertonicity:	overtightness or overcontraction of muscle or tendon tissue
hypertrophy:	growth of tissue from use
inflammation:	the reaction of vascularized living tissue to local injury, involving a series of changes that occur as the body repairs itself and replaces damaged or dead tissue with healthy tissue.
ipsilateral:	on the same side of the body
lateral:	away from the midline of the body (toward the sides)
ligament:	fibrous, collagenous tissue connecting bone to bone
medial:	toward the midline of the body
nerve plexus:	a network of nerves arising from the spinal segments
neuritis:	inflammation of a nerve
palmar:	palm side of the hand in anatomical position

paresthesias: numbness and tingling

posterior: pertaining to the back of the body

prodrome: physiologic changes and symptoms that precede the full expression of a disorder

prone: a position in which the individual lies face down, on her stomach

radial deviation: movement of the hand at the wrist in the direction of the radius

referred pain: pain that is felt at a site other than its origin

scar tissue: connective tissue that replaces original tissue damaged by trauma at an injury site

sign: objective evidence of illness or dysfunction (as opposed to *symptom*)

sprain: a condition involving complete or partial tearing of ligamentous tissue

strain: a condition involving complete or partial tearing of muscle or tendon tissue

subclinical: changes due to injury or disease that cannot be consciously perceived

supine: a position in which the individual lies face up, on her back

symptom: subjective evidence of illness or dysfunction

syndrome: a group of symptoms or signs related to each other by some physiologic abnormality

systemic: affecting the entire body

tendon: tissue connecting muscle to bone. Combination of mostly fibrous tissue with some elastic tissue.

ulnar deviation: movement of the hand at the wrist in the direction of the ulna

volar: pertaining to the palm side of the forearm

Appendix IV
Bibliography

The following books were used in my research. I highly recommend them to any massage therapist who would like to understand more about injury physiology, prevention, and treatment.

Anderson, Bob. *Stretching*. Bolinas, California: Shelter Publications, Inc., 1980.

Ashley, Martin. *Massage: A Career At Your Fingertips*. Barrytown, New York: Station Hill Press, Inc., 1992.

Benjamin, Ben E., with Borden, Gale. *Listen To Your Pain*. New York: Penguin Books, 1984.

Butler, David. *Mobilization of the Nervous System*. Churchilll Livingston, 1991.

Cailliet, Rene. *Hand Pain and Impairment*. Philadelphia: F.A. Davis Company, 1982.

Cailliet, Rene. *Soft Tissue Pain and Dysfunction*. Philadelphia: F.A. Davis Company, 1991.

Chaitow, Leon. *Soft-Tissue Manipulation*. Rochester, VT: Healing Arts Press, 1980.

Evans, Maja. *The Ultimate Hand Book*. Laughing Duck Press, 1992.

Feldenkrais, Moshe. *Awareness Through Movement*. San Francisco: Harper, 1990.

Gray, John. *The Alexander Technique*. New York: St. Martin's Press, 1990.

Jenkins, David B. *Hollinshead's Functional Anatomy of the Limbs and Back*. W.B. Saunders Company, 1991.

Juhan, Deane. *Job's Body*. Barrytown, New York: Station Hill Press, 1987.

Kahle, W., Leonhardt, H., and Platzer, W. *Color Atlas and Textbook of Human Anatomy: Locomotor System*. Stuttgart-New York: Georg Thieme Verlag, 1986.

Pascarelli, Emil and Quilter, Deborah. *Repetitive Strain Injury*. New York: John Wiley & Sons, Inc., 1994.

Sellers, Don. *ZAP! How your computer can hurt you - and what you can do about it*. Berkeley, California: Peachpit Press, 1994.

Tappan, Frances M. *Healing Massage Techniques*: *Holistic, Classic and Emerging Methods*. Appleton & Lange, 1988.

Thomas, Clayton L. (ed.). *Taber's Cyclopedic Medical Dictionary* (17th ed.). Philadelphia, PA: F.A. Davis Co., 1993.

Thompson, Diana L. *Hands Heal: Documentation for Massage Therapy*. Seattle, Washington: Diana L. Thompson, 1993.

Tortora, Gerard J. *Principles of Anatomy*. New York: Harper Collins Publishers, 1989.

Index

ABOUT THE AUTHOR

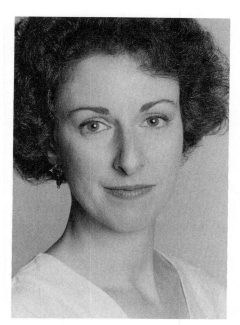

Lauriann Greene, L.M.P., graduated with honors from Seattle Massage School and has been a teaching assistant and tutor for the school. She studied previously at Brown and Harvard Universities, and attended the Mannes College of Music in New York City, her hometown. As a former professional orchestral conductor and pianist, Ms. Greene was interested in working with other musicians to reduce playing-related upper extremity injury. This interest led her to write and publish an article on musicians' injuries that appeared in the Spring, 1994 issue of *Massage Therapy Journal* (featuring Ms. Greene on the cover). Research from that article and her own experience with massage-related wrist injury led Ms. Greene to develop the *"Save Your Hands!"* workshops for massage therapists. She began teaching the workshops at Seattle Massage School's three campuses in 1993. Since that time, she has taught injury prevention to massage therapy students and professionals in Vancouver, British Columbia and across the United States. Ms. Greene resides in Seattle, Washington and remains active as a performing musician and dancer, writer, and editor.